George Michael's

COMPLETE
HAIR CARE
FOR MEN

George Michael's

COMPLETE HAIR CARE FOR MEN

by George Michael
and Rae Lindsay

Doubleday & Company, Inc.
Garden City, New York
1983

Photos of George Michael courtesy of Wagner International Photos. Drawings and all other photos courtesy of Pivot Point International.

Design by Beverley Vawter Gallegos

Library of Congress Cataloging in Publication Data
Michael, George, 1918–
George Michael's complete hair care for men.
Includes index.
1. Hair—Care and hygiene.   2. Grooming for
men.   I. Lindsay, Rae.   II. Title.
RL91.M5   1983   646.7'24'088041   AACR2
ISBN 0-385-17450-0
Library of Congress Catalog Card Number 82–45114

To all the men whose women have been my patrons

and to all my associates

in the wonderful hairdressing profession

for the past quarter century.

Acknowledgments

My thanks and love to Maria Rae Lindsay who once again worked with me devotedly and effectively in creating this book.

Special thanks to Leo Passage, president of Pivot Point International, for his assistance in providing photographic material and other illustrations.

Contents

Introduction

The Samson Syndrome—
Traditions, Theories and Trends
About Men and Their Hair

Hair is one of a man's prized possessions; it is a mark of personal identity, a sex symbol, a frame for his face, an indication of status, class and even age. Hair is as important to a man's image as the clothes he wears and the way he talks.

Given the crucial role hair plays in how a man looks, it's remarkable that in our century, until the last decade anyway, men always associated too much attention to their looks with a lack of masculinity. The idea was always that if a man worried or cared about the health or appearance of his hair or skin he was foppish, or effeminate.

This conclusion has always seemed rather strange to me, because when you look at the big picture, hair and strength have gone together during most of recorded history. Think of Samson, the strongest man in the world. As the Bible tells us, he had a mass of hair, and unquestioned strength and virility, until he lost his hair and his head over Delilah. Jesus Christ had long hair, and so did his disciples. Can you visualize Robin Hood or Lancelot with a crew cut? Was Charlemagne bald? Hair was so important to America's founding fathers that if they didn't have it, they wore wigs, as did George Washington and Thomas Jefferson. And English judges still wear powdered wigs as a symbol of the power of justice.

But the first short hairstyles for men started with Alexander the Great of Macedon, way back in 336 B.C., when he had all his soldiers' hair cut short (and their beards shaved) so they would be less vulnerable in hand-to-hand combat. With no beards and short hair, enemies were robbed of a convenient handhold and a source for inflicting pain. Alexander conquered the world, so presumably there was some merit to his philosophy. Then too, short hair reduced the incidence of lice and other hygiene problems prevalent when men are living in a communal situation.

Very short hair also robs a man of a measure of personal identity, the individual variations that make a man look uniquely like himself and nobody else. Taking their cue from Alexander the Great, through time men entering military service or prison have had their hair cut very short. In any kind of institution it's easier to maintain discipline and order when identity and individuality are suppressed, and a haircut like everyone else's effectively achieves this universality.

After Alexander, the long hair and short hair customs took turns in popularity right up until modern history. During the Dark Ages, for example, if a nobleman grew really long hair, dictatorial clergymen might make him cut his hair off publicly to teach him a moral lesson about vanity and masculine strength. It was a disgrace for men to have long hair, but a glory for women. (Lady Godiva comes to mind as the female side of the coin for this period.)

A similar attitude about hair was graphically expressed a few centuries later in Russia, around the end of the seventeenth century, when Tsar Peter the Great decided all noblemen should look like the shorn Samson. He would ask the gentlemen of his court to visit him and with a huge pair of scissors in hand he would personally cut off feet of hair which had been cherished for years, and he would lop off beards that had grown to the chest or longer. Kindly, he would give his victims a little shot of vodka after the shearing to make the loss somewhat easier to take.

These were the practices that eventually brainwashed men about their hair. Long hair is for women, mystics or rock singers or homosexuals; short hair is for *real* men. All these clichés were blasted by the hippies of a decade ago, and although their own ponytails and shoulder-length curls are passé today, they did achieve a breakthrough in how men felt about and treated and cared for their hair.

There is still some resistance, however, and too many men still think that serious emphasis on hair is unmasculine. Even though men don't wear crew cuts today, even though they now have their hair "styled" instead of cut, I still see this negative approach when a man comes to me for a consultation, always because he's *losing* his hair. When a woman is troubled by hair loss she always comes right to the point: "Mr. Michael—my hair is falling out! What can I do? Help me!"

The man comes in and spends forty-five minutes talking about how virile he is. He wants me to know he's not vain, that he is not a sissy worried about something frivolous like losing his hair. It's not frivolous or sissyish to worry about losing your hair; the man who *doesn't* admit to this kind of concern is the one who is denying his own masculinity.

Certainly most men lose their hair through hereditary pattern baldness, but a good many men have hair fallout problems because of "benign neglect": they simply don't know how to take care of their hair and haven't bothered to learn because of those old clichés about what's macho and what's not. There's another problem here, too. Now that men are wearing their hair longer, bleaching it, dyeing it, using blowdryers, hair sprays, thickeners and other commercial products they are experiencing fallout caused by abuse. They don't know what they're using nor what they are doing.

Another major problem with men and their hair is that from the earliest years on they have a kind of "me, too" acceptance about hair care and hair loss. It reminds me of the three-year-old boy who says, "I'm a meat-and-potatoes man," just because his father is a meat-and-potatoes man. But what does he know? If you give him chicken or lobster tomorrow, he'll probably become a "chicken-or-lobster man." Children imitate what they see and hear, and just as he wants to eat as his father does, he'll follow his father's habits of hair care, for better or worse.

When he grows up, he switches from father's influence to barber's influence. It's traditional for many men to go to the barber, ask him to "take a little off around the ears," close their eyes and have a nap while the barber does exactly what he feels like doing. Although most barbers now call themselves stylists, the decision making about that haircut is often still left up to the person who doesn't own that head of hair.

Whether the reason is conditioning and/or training, men just don't know enough about their hair to care for it optimally. You have to understand, to begin with, that your hair is different from your wife's or girl's hair. First off, her hair is *better* because it's the secretion of female hormones that produces hair on the head, and women secrete more female hormones. One reason doctors haven't been able to come up with a cure for baldness is that if they give men excessive female hormones men will develop breasts and acquire other feminizing physical traits.

You also have to understand that the products and techniques your lady uses or recommends aren't necessarily right for you—just as your father's techniques were not necessarily right for you. The way she brushes or shampoos or conditions her hair may, in fact, be *wrong* for you.

This is the time to think about you and your hair and to find out what works best for you, to drop old habits, misconceptions and hang-ups and enjoy results that are based on the truth of your situation, not somebody else's hand-me-down ideas or rituals.

My goal in this book is to provide you with all the ammunition and know-how you need to have the best-looking hair and keep it that way. This is not a book about hairstyling alone; nor is it merely a book on baldness and how to cope with it. Both these subjects are covered, along with much more. What we will present to you in the following pages is the first complete hair care book for men, a book that spells out in step-by-step detail what you *can* do to encourage and maintain the best hair *you* can have; what you *can't* do in terms of limitations imposed by hormones, heredity and other given factors; and finally, what you *can* do to get around such givens via hair transplants and other techniques.

The major emphasis, of course, is prevention and maintenance, and these are tied in with knowledge: knowledge of how to take care of your hair—what to eat, how to massage, how to shampoo; knowledge of which conditioners can achieve body and control; knowledge of the styles that suit your face and your life.

I always tell the thirty-six thousand clients who have come to my salon during the past two decades that hair doesn't have to be their worst enemy . . . that if they follow my guidelines and adopt my techniques and rules, hair can become their best friend. My aim is to accomplish the same results for you in this first book on hair care specifically written for men.

PART ONE

How to Make the Most of the Hair You Inherited

Chapter One

Physical Exercise, Massage and Brushing

The health, strength and even abundance of your hair is directly dependent upon how much exercise you and your scalp get.

In this sense women have a distinct advantage over men because they have been taught from the time they were old enough to hold a brush to wield the proverbial hundred strokes every day—and this becomes a natural massage. Did you ever know a man who did this? (Actually, men shouldn't brush a hundred strokes unless their hair is in really excellent condition. Twenty-five to thirty strokes is more than adequate.) In addition, women comb their hair often during the day, which can be another form of massage. Most men look in the mirror in the morning, comb or brush their hair so it's groomed, and that's that, unless they're caught in a hurricane during their lunch hour. (There's a trade-off here, though, because when men shave every morning they are enjoying a natural skin massage and getting rid of dead surface cells in a way women can't imitate.)

Basically, though, the health of your hair is directly related to the state of your blood circulation. If blood flow is poor, this can cause a great many problems, including abnormal fallout. While the *quality* of the blood counts (and this is determined by the quality of your eating habits), it is essential that sufficient *quantities* of blood reach the roots to feed the hair cell at the site of its formation. You can increase the rate of circulation to your scalp in three ways: through exercise, through massage, and by proper brushing.

Exercise Requisites

Men in certain occupations get more natural exercise than those in other professions, and this can contribute to hair loss caused by other than hereditary conditions. An accountant, for example, only exercises his fingers when he works a calculator, but a farmer or a longshoreman exercises his legs, his arms, his chest muscles. He will naturally have better hair as well as a better body.

Sports, of course, are good for the entire body, but such vigorous exercises as tennis or racquetball may backfire because after a strenuous hour on the courts you may be very hungry or thirsty and will eat or drink more than you should, canceling out the weight-maintenance aspects of the sport. In addition, many busy executives cannot devote themselves to two- or three-hour-long (or longer) sessions necessary to be skillful at a sport, and more important, the time required for this sport to really aid the body. I personally find myself in this position. My work involves a heavy and erratic schedule; there is no way I can arrange to play tennis at such and such a time each week. But there are other exercises I can arrange at my own time, that I can engage in wherever I am—in any part of the world—that not only keep my body well toned and keep the circulation moving, but also afford me peace of mind and relaxation. These exercises are walking and yoga.

For years I've believed that walking beats jogging any day in terms of overall benefits, so I'm glad to see that recent medical research bears out my opinion. When you walk you're not straining any muscles or other part of your body, and you're using your legs and arms in a natural movement, unlike the heel-toe movements of jogging, which place undue stress on the vulnerable and overworked foot, and actually do not provide exercise benefits for the arms and torso—although jogging, like walking, is excellent for exercising the heart. I live right across from Central Park in New York, and after a day's work (or sometimes before my workday begins) there's nothing nicer than a brisk walk in the park when I can either relax my mind after twelve hours of chaos . . . or prepare myself for the day ahead.

Wherever I am, whether on a beach in St. Thomas or getting ready to address a meeting of five hundred doctors and trichologists in Switzerland, I always find an hour to take a good long walk.

The other form of exercise I recommend is yoga—the asanas, or postures, which are quite different from the actual practice of yoga, which is more a question of learning to relax through meditation and concentration. This isn't the place to go into yoga in depth, but in terms of circulation and all-over bodily health, it would be a good idea to learn how to do a headstand, or a modified headstand (in which your legs are not straight up but bent in a manner that's an easier balance for beginners), or even a shoulder stand.

Yoga asanas are also marvelous for working on specific body areas in a nonstrenuous way. For our purposes, here are two yoga routines which encourage circulation to the scalp while relaxing tension in the head and neck areas.

The Neck Roll

1. Sit in a crossed-legged posture.

2. Bend your head forward slowly and rest your chin against your chest. Be sure to sit erect.

3. Close eyes and hold this position for a count of ten.

4. Very slowly roll head to the extreme left. Don't move the trunk of your body. Sit erect. Hold for a count of ten.

5. Very slowly roll head to extreme backward position. You'll feel your chin and throat muscles tightening. Hold for a count of ten.

6. Slowly roll head to extreme right. Keep body erect. Hold for a count of ten.

7. Very slowly roll head forward so that your chin rests on your chest. Don't move your trunk. Hold for a count of ten.

8. Relax for a few seconds; repeat routine two more times.

The Head Twist

1. Lie on your stomach; plant elbows on the floor. Put your head between your hands and close your eyes.

2. Slowly push your head downward with your hands until your chin touches your chest. Hold for a count of ten.

3. Raise your head, place chin in right palm and place left hand firmly on the back of your head (your elbows remain on the floor). Slowly twist head to the right. Hold for a count of ten.

4. Turn head frontward; place chin in left palm and place your right hand on the back of your head. Very slowly twist to the left and hold for a count of ten.

5. Turn head frontward; relax; repeat routine once more.

The Massage Message

While men will do anything, learn anything, that will make them shine in their professions, when it comes to their hair, often they operate on a premise of *que será será* or engage in what my psychiatrist friends call crisis intervention. In other words, either they adopt an attitude of "what will be, will be," or when the hair fallout is reaching disaster proportions, then they will try to do something to correct it, or stem the tide of baldness.

This attitude carries over to massage. Many men feel that if a little bit helps, a lot more will help a lot more and are inclined to be very gung ho when I tell them to massage their scalps. There's a misconception that stronger is better. This isn't so. A very enthusiastic massage will tell you your scalp is alive, but in the meantime, if you work your hands through your hair energetically, you're also ripping off half of the hair.

If a man is still holding on to his crew cut, fine; he can do this without harming his hair. But if the hair is four to six inches in length, he's much better off using a gentler technique of massage. I have a special prescription for my friends—men and women alike—who are doctors or psychiatrists or lawyers who have to sit in a chair for hours listening to patients or clients. Between appointments I recommend that they sit with their heads between their knees, elbows hanging down and fingertips spread over the forehead and scalp (thumbs at the temples), and massage up and down very slowly, about thirty movements per sixty seconds, and continue this massage for one minute. If this can be repeated ten times a day, scalp condition, and subsequently hair condition, will improve almost immediately.

If you doubt the merits of massage, put your fingers on your scalp and using the tip of each index finger, gently move your scalp. It seems firm, tight, uncooperative. Now move your fingers in a circular motion and see how your scalp responds—almost like a dog you've petted for a few seconds.

There are two types of massage: the kind you give yourself, and the kind another person can do for you. The latter, of course, is more satisfying because that brings with it the fact that someone else is kind enough and committed enough to provide the loving touch of massage. So we'll give you both ways, which you can enjoy according to your social or marital, or whatever situation.

Do-It-Yourself Scalp Massage

Lie on your bed with your head hanging over the edge. Place your hands, fingers spread open, so that your thumbs are above your ears and your little fingers meet at the top of your forehead. Then, moving your fingers in an up-and-down "regrasping" motion, massage about twenty times in this position. Move on to the next position an inch or so higher on your head and repeat (your thumbs may still be in the same place above your ears). Move on again toward the back of your head (by now your thumbs are farther down behind your ears). Continue until you've covered the entire head.

Although this massage in a heads-down position makes optimum chances for improved circulation, if you do this sitting up—at your desk, watching television, waiting for a traffic light to change—you'll still be passing on great benefits to your scalp and hair. If your hair is normal to dry, repeat this at least once a day; if you have oily hair, massage only two or three times a week.

Massage with a Willing Partner

While you lie down on your back, she stands or kneels behind you and gently but firmly lifts your head in her hands. Make sure she's doing the lifting and not you. Then she slowly rotates your head in a *clockwise* movement, returning to the original lift position, and repeats once more.

Next, she holds your head in place for five seconds, then rotates it twice in a *counterclockwise* position. This step of the massage is completed when she glides her hands down over the sides of your neck and onto your shoulders.

Step Two Massage—"Brushing the Forehead"

She rests her fingers at your temples and centers her thumbs at the middle of your forehead, up at the hairline. She will use a very light pressure, brushing her thumbs out toward her fingers, returning with an even lighter pressure to the center of the forehead and repeating the brushstroke, beginning at a slightly lower point each time until the entire area from the hairline to the brow bone is massaged.

Step Three Massage—"The Temple Relaxer"

Starting at the temples, she rotates the first three fingers of each hand in small circles going outward toward the hair. Beginning at the top of the temples, she works all the way around them and over the natural temple depression. She should continue this movement, working downward until she comes to the top of the cheekbone. At this point, she uses the first two fingers to glide back upward from the cheekbones to the top of the temples. She should repeat these motions once more.

And incidentally, when she finishes, you should return the favor.

What to Use, When and How to Brush Your Hair

Not only do you have to know *how* to brush, but it's important to know *what kind* of brush to use. Men are very casual about the kind of brush they buy to groom their hair, and this is another example of misinformation. A man's brush is very different from a woman's. If she has hair more than six inches long, she should use a brush that's semiround, which encourages a rotating motion of the wrist. Of course, if you have hair that long or longer, you should use the same type of brush.

But if your hair is four to six inches long, you should use a "club" brush, a flat brush which can be used in a flat motion all around your head without rotating your wrist.

There are brushes and brushes, and natural bristle brushes of all price ranges, just as there are cars and cars. The Rolls-Royce, Eldorado convertible, Mercedes-Benz of brushes is made by Kent of London to my specifications. I'll be telling you more about these brushes in Chapter Five.

It's important to know when to brush your hair, too. And my rule is, brush your hair in the morning. When you go to bed at night, your body is in a horizontal position and the blood circulation is actually concentrated toward the scalp. Then, when you get up in the morning, the blood rushes from your head and down to your legs, which can even make you feel dizzy. For this reason, it's never a good idea to spring up from bed as soon as the alarm goes off. After your wake-up time, lie in bed for a few minutes. First stretch your arms, then your legs, then all of your limbs together. Did you ever see the way a cat or dog wakes up? Animals wake up in stages, never abruptly. Would you run your car at seventy miles an hour immediately after switching on the ignition? No, you give it a chance to warm up.

During the day your body is active and blood, if you're healthy, is circulating all through your body. Therefore, nighttime brushing, while it can be very sexy when a woman brushes her hair, only adds a little to the circulation that has been going on for most of the day. In the morning you have to even out that quick rush of blood to your limbs by restoring circulation to the scalp.

Don't brush your hair as if you were trying to eliminate your worst enemy. This procedure is really a favor to a friend of yours, your hair. So you brush slowly to avoid tensing up the scalp muscles; brushing should be relaxing for the muscles and at the same time stimulating for the circulation. Remember, too, that brushing helps distribute the beneficial fats and oils of the scalp to encourage a shine, even if it's not coming from a healthy, transparent hair cuticle. It's most important, however, to realize that brushing *does* stimulate the growth and health of the hair roots, and this is essential for the all-over condition of your hair.

If, however, your hair is in an *unhealthy* condition—if you are suffering from stress, infection, hormone problems, any of numerous reasons for excessive fallout that we'll be talking about later—then brushing will rush the departure of those hairs, which have now been programmed to leave anyway. In other words, if your hair is in bad condition for any one of many reasons, the avoidance of brushing will not cure the problem; it will merely make you *think* you have arrested it.

Chapter Two

Keep It Clean—
When, What, How to Shampoo

If you get your hair wet in the shower every day, that counts as a shampoo, right? Wrong! Yet many men think that a daily wet-down does the trick. Although men have been washing their own hair from the time they were six or seven, nobody ever taught them how to do it properly.

Often a man will reach for whatever shampoo happens to be in the tub or shower—whatever his wife, or girl, or teenage daughter stashes there. And this shampoo may be perfect for them, but not for him.

We're not really talking about shampoo for the hair as much as selecting the right product for the scalp and the hair roots. Hair is dead, the scalp and roots are alive, and these are the crucial factors in making a decision. There's been a lot of confusing talk recently about "the pH factor," and "the acid mantle," and whether a product is acid or alkaline. To erase some confusion about this very important aspect of hair (and, as a matter of fact, skin, because your scalp is after all, skin), these are the facts:

The pH range is 0 to 7, acid; 7 to 14, alkaline. The most neutral acid/alkaline condition is 7. Pure water is always 7, for example. While, generally, most hair is 4.6 (on the acid side, like Pepsi-Cola or Coca-Cola), the most important numbers of all never change. They are the same for everybody. The key figure is 2.6 for the extremely acid hair roots; the second number to remember is 5.6, the pH factor for everyone's scalp. (The reason the hair itself is less acid and actually varies from the 4.6 average is oxidation, which changes the chemical structure of the hair strands which have been exposed to the elements.)

A simpler way of explaining the pH factor is to realize that hair roots are living things, like a fish or a human. A fish lives in water, a human lives in the air. You have to put hair where it lives. If you take a man out of the air and put him in the water, he will die; if you take a fish out of water and put it in the air, it will die. You have to keep hair in its most viable environment.

This seems very sensible and logical, and yet I'm constantly amazed that people who should know better actually knock the hell out of their hair. A few months ago a doctor friend came to see me. He is about forty and experiencing a great deal of trauma over his increasing baldness. I looked at his scalp and asked him, "What kind of shampoo do you use?" I couldn't believe his answer: "tincture of green soap." Shocked, I asked him why and he said, "Well, when I was a resident I couldn't afford to buy shampoo and I knew tincture of green soap was good for scrubbing up (before surgery), and I've used it ever since."

Of course he knew that *tincture* means an alcohol or alkaline base, as opposed to a solution, which means a water base but he continued using it anyway. By using alcohol he was actually robbing his hair of any natural fat. In a sense he was *dry cleaning* his hair constantly. No wonder it was falling out!

There is a very simple rule about shampoos that men and women of all ages should learn: you have to put back what you take out of your hair. The solution is not to find a shampoo that's 2.6 or even one that is 5.6, because neither of these will lather enough to do a cleansing job, but to find one that is somewhere between the 8 pH you need for adequate lather to cleanse externally and the 2.6 pH you need to restore the acidity of your hair roots.

It's true, though, that long or short, everyone with hair is looking for that special shampoo, that miracle worker to make hair sparkle, bounce, look *wonderful.* And of course, with the barrage of advertising in magazines, radio, television, we are tempted to keep trying and buying. This leads to a lot of fads—in fact, just about every season there is a new shampoo fad.

Protein—Plus or Minus?

One of the longest-lasting and most highly touted gimmicks, not only for shampoo but in fact for every hair care product from conditioners to sprays, is *protein,* possibly the most overused word in the beauty industry.

Remember that no matter what you rub on your hair or skin, it simply will not become part of the hair itself. The substance may lie there on the surface and seemingly improve the appearance or texture of the hair, but it doesn't actually do anything intrinsic to better the quality of your hair. The only way you can get deep-down protein benefits is if you eat protein and then your liver, the body's nuclear reactor, splits these proteins into absorbable elements that will actually benefit your hair roots and scalp.

Among the protein-enriched shampoos have been those that include eggs and/or milk as "magic" ingredients. I have found through my testing that the addition of eggs or milk often does more harm than good, because after repeated use the substances just "sit" on the hair, coating it in a way that interferes with shine and manageability.

Still, dozens of new shampoos are introduced each year, all basing their claim to fame on a gimmick. After the egg shampoo and the milk shampoo, we had a whole range of herbal shampoos, fruit shampoos, lemon shampoos. There are smelly gimmicks, tasty gimmicks, scientific gimmicks, beautiful gimmicks. But they are just that: gimmicks.

You must keep in mind that shampoo is ultimately only an agent. It doesn't speak English, it doesn't talk to you. Its only job is to cleanse your hair and maintain the health and appearance of your hair while it's cleansing. Although I might recommend a very expensive hair-brush, I would never insist that you buy expensive shampoo. This would be outrageous because the hair stays on your head (and you need a good brush to keep it there), but the shampoo goes down the drain.

I have spent more than two decades testing various shampoos; many were terrible, some were quite good, and others reached a level of performance that was close to my own standards. But not quite close enough. After years of research I have been able to develop my own line of hair care products for men and women, and although this sounds self-serving, the important fact is that hair behaves better and looks better when these products are used in conjunction with my specific rules and regulations for hair care. The products I recommend are cream shampoos for coarse hair and liquid shampoos for fine, limp hair.

How to Shampoo

The word shampoo comes from the ancient Hindu and means *massage*. The implication here is that you don't just plunk half a bottle of shampoo on your head, rub it in vigorously as if you were attacking an enemy and rinse it off. A good shampoo has a twofold effect: (1) it cleanses the hair and (2) it provides a gentle massage that calms and relaxes your head while increasing circulation to the scalp—a boon for healthy hair. But the key word is *gentle*. Here's how to shampoo your hair the right way—one of those things Mother (or Dad) never told you.

For the first sudsing, the goal is to remove all superfluous particles of dirt and oil from the scalp. If you're using a good nondetergent shampoo you will not have much lather on the first sudsing. (In fact, if you do have lather, you know you're using a detergent shampoo.) This first sudsing is simply to slosh off the dirt. During your second lathering you'll be massaging your scalp—not your hair. For the correct massage, first work around the hairline, moving your hands toward the crown and massaging the scalp; then work your fingers up from the nape of your neck to the top of your head and shampoo the scalp in up and down motions. Don't use the hair itself as a scrub brush. Just make sure you massage the shampoo into your entire scalp; it should feel loose, pliable, relaxed.

After the shampoo make sure you've really rinsed your hair thoroughly with lukewarm water, and then, to give your hair more body (a pickup for the rest of your body, too), finish off with a cool to cold last rinse. The cold water shrinks the molecules of the hair and knocks off any superfluous coatings, making your hair much more manageable. If you're reading this book in the winter, don't start rinsing with cold water immediately; it will be too shocking. But in any other season when the weather is still fairly mild, adopt a program of rinsing your hair first with warm, then lukewarm and finally cold water.

It's important to get your body accustomed to changes in temperature, whether of the air or of the water. One of my grandmother's sisters was a midwife in Russia and was considered the neighborhood madcap because of her penchant for swimming every day, all year long. In the middle of winter she would take a big ice pick to the river, chop out a small swimming hole, and dip herself in the water for about ten minutes. Even in her mid-seventies, this was a daily habit. People wondered how she could do it, but the answer was simple. If she tried it the first time in the middle of winter, she would have died of pneumonia, but the fact that it was her everyday routine meant that her body had been gradually conditioned to the icy water.

How Often to Shampoo

While theoretically you could shampoo every hour with the proper product, how often you actually do shampoo depends on many factors —your life-style, whether your scalp is oily or not, the season. In summer, for example, your hair gets dirtier because you perspire more. If you wear hats outdoors in winter or summer, your hair will stay cleaner. If you cook a lot or smoke a great deal you may want to wash your hair more often to eliminate odors that accumulate in the hair. On the other hand, a patient going into the hospital for surgery may not have to worry about shampooing his hair for several weeks because he won't be exposed to pollution or normal day-to-day soil. Basically, hair of any length should be washed only as often as necessary. Too much shampooing dries out the hair, although it doesn't affect the hair root at all. Hair is lost not by *washing* but by strenuous scrubbing!

Dandruff Is a Disaster

From the time you were a kid you've been inundated by those commercials warning against the social failings of those "telltale flakes." These, of course, were designed to make you buy *that* particular product. But dandruff is not something anybody should dismiss as just another advertising ploy to get you to buy a certain shampoo. Dandruff is actually an infectious, annoying and possibly contagious disease. Medically, dandruff is identified as pityriasis, and it is characterized by continued, excessive shedding of dead, "cornified" cells from the scalp. Problems with dandruff usually begin during adolescence and reach a peak in the early twenties. Those annoying "telltale" flakes are often more apparent and severe in the winter months in temperate climates. Although dandruff may be contagious (sufferers should be very careful about lending their brushes, combs or other hair implements), it can be controlled rather effectively (although not eliminated) with special shampoos.

Any ordinary nonmedicated soap or shampoo will remove the surface flakes from the scalp as they form, but specially formulated antidandruff shampoos actually work to keep the disease at bay, rather than simply eliminating the symptoms. One of the best antidandruff agents I've come across (also recommended by medical authorities) is

Breck One, formerly called Breck Banish, which contains zinc pyrithione. This chemical is also found in such shampoos as Head & Shoulders, Zincon and Danex. Another chemical, selenium sulfide, used in Selsun, Selsun Blue and others, also works well against dandruff. Selsun has developed a new conditioner, Selene, which helps to restore the balance and pliability of the hair (disturbed by other shampoos).

A third group of shampoos contains coal tar, which has also been found to be a good dandruff deterrent. In this last case I feel the results are less cosmetically acceptable (the hair has an unpleasant smell after shampooing); in addition, such products are somewhat harsh and strip away the natural hair oils while getting rid of the dandruff.

Watch the Water

No matter how careful you are about which shampoo you use and how you shampoo, if you live in an area with hard water, the increased quantity of mineral deposits can be damaging. It may be necessary to "soften" the water by adding a few drops of cream rinse or a commercial water softener to a quart of water and use this as a final rinse after shampooing.

This practice is especially helpful in the Midwest and in mountainous areas where water has a tremendous amount of iron. New Yorkers should stop cursing their water because it's among the best in the country. Visitors often comment on how good the tea and coffee taste. I've always maintained that we have excellent water here in New York City, so I was amused some months ago when one of the television stations did a taste test on various bottled waters and New York's own. The plain old free-from-the-tap variety outshone four or five costly, chic bottled waters. In fact, Macy's began to sell New York water as a specialty item in their gourmet shop. New York water not only tastes good, but it's wonderful for your hair!

Chapter Three

A Seminar in Management— How to Keep Your Hair in Top Condition

By now some of the pieces of the puzzle are falling into place. You know how to brush and massage to increase circulation, and how to keep your hair clean. But don't quit now, because you only know about a quarter of the story.

All of the knowledge you've acquired so far won't help you keep your hair under control and/or in optimum condition. While you're doing all these things correctly, nature and the environment and even your own heredity may be working against you. There's no question that all of us suffer a lot of abuse to our bodies and our hair because of the world we live in—as well as the world we make.

Fortunately, our bodies are wonderfully designed mechanisms that have built-in adjustments for such natural or unnatural stresses. And so does our hair. The fragile, delicate appearance of a strand of hair is totally deceptive. Hair is actually so strong that if you exposed it to air indefinitely, it would survive for 680 years.

If you took that same piece of hair and placed it in an airtight container with a controlled temperature between 40 and 80 degrees and a humidity level between 56 and 75 percent, the hair would not disintegrate for eight to ten thousand years!

This is a nice bit of scientific trivia, illustrated, as a matter of fact, by the recent discovery of the mummified remains of a Chinese noble-woman who still had a full head of hair after being buried for more than three thousand years. However, it's useful only as trivia because your hair, my hair, everybody's hair, suffers from our space-age environment and other abuses, most of them self-inflicted. Our air is polluted, often the water we drink and wash with is laden with chemicals, the hair is pulled, stretched, dried, drowned, frozen, overheated, ignored or drenched with attention. With all these assaults, we can't expect hair to survive for a lifetime, much less the long-term endurance trials mentioned above.

We do a lot to our hair and take a lot out of it, all of which has to be put back. The ideal way, of course, is from the inside, via your diet, as will be explained in Chapter Eleven. But this chapter is about the *external* ways you can bring your hair back to healthy life and keep it that way through what is known in my trade as *conditioning*.

Let me explain conditioning in terms of other professions. If you own an expensive IBM word processor you know that you'll get the best results out of that equipment if you have it serviced regularly, as opposed to waiting until the machine breaks down. This kind of attention is also true for your car, or should be. In the field of medicine, more and more emphasis is being put on annual checkups and tests to nip any problems in the bud, rather than having to deal with a *fait accompli*. The operative word in all these examples is *prevention*.

Conditioning is precisely that: preventive medicine. By taking appropriate care of your hair on an ongoing basis, using simple techniques and readily available commercial products, you can ward off disasters and maintain the best-looking head of hair possible.

Seasonal Switches

It would be convenient for all of us if I could say, "Take this bottle of XYZ, apply it to your hair all year long and you've got it made." But I can't unless you happen to live in a climate that stays the same 365 days a year, like the tropics. Just as you need different kinds of clothing for different seasons, you need to vary the products and care you use on your hair in keeping with weather and temperature changes. It's important to realize that your hair changes with the temperature. In the wintertime hair molecules shrink and you can use an emulsion-type conditioner that works in a short amount of time—for example, my conditioner which is left on for sixty seconds.

In the summertime, hair molecules are in an extremely expanded state, the hair actually swells and requires a slower-acting, cream-type conditioner which is left on for ten or twelve minutes.

Now even this sounds simple enough: one type of conditioner for hot weather; another for cold weather. But a common failing, shared by men and women, is that if a little bit helps, a lot more will help a lot more. Don't make the mistake of overdoing a good thing. Too much conditioning (except when you're swimming) results in a buildup of residue that detracts from the health of your hair. In most cases, once-a-month home conditioning will do the trick. Curly hair, which is very porous and reacts so frizzily to humidity, may require more frequent conditioning. Naturally, you only condition *clean* hair, just as you never apply a coat of touch-up paint to a boat or a room that's dirty.

Another caution: it's not enough to schedule regular conditioning and let it go at that. You have to combine the use of these products with some protective measures especially dictated by the seasons.

Winter Problems

If I ask ten people which is the most ruinous season for hair, summer or winter, nine out of ten will say summer—and nine out of ten will be wrong. Winter does the most damage to hair because we are constantly going from one environment to another. At home or in your office, to save energy, you keep the thermostat set at 68 degrees, and your utility company thanks you, the President of the United States thanks you and I thank you. Then you rush out for a business appointment, you can't get a bus or subway, so you walk for fifteen minutes in 15-degree weather. Your mother would love your nice rosy cheeks (you're her little boy again) and laugh at your nice red ears. Of course your hair doesn't feel cold—it's dead—but your scalp is freezing if you're the type of man who habitually refuses to wear hats.

Then, during your meeting, you're in agony because although the temperature is hovering around 72, there is no air in the room and the tweed suit, suede vest and wool socks are as uncomfortable for you as the proverbial hair shirt. That change from hot to cold to even hotter makes your hair expand and shrink and expand violently. Not only do you catch cold with these shifts in temperature, but you subject your hair to extremes never undergone by that sheltered three-thousand-year-old mummy we talked about earlier. Incidentally, this doesn't happen in the summertime because the difference between shade and sun is only about 17 degrees, and even if you go from an air-conditioned environment to the natural, hot outdoors, you're only talking about a relatively small contrast in temperature.

Despite the energy crisis, not only do too many stores, offices and other commercial businesses keep the thermostat turned up too high during the winter, but artificial heating (and, as a matter of record, air conditioning) rob the atmosphere of humidity and the result is that your scalp and your skin get dried out (47 percent humidity is ideal for good health and good hair).

A room humidifier helps in summer *or* winter; even placing a pan of water near a radiator adds humidity to a room which your skin and your plants will be grateful for. Your records will last longer and your dog will love the improved atmosphere, too. About once a week, it's also a good idea to enjoy the humidity produced by your washing machine or dishwasher. Just open the door for a few minutes while it's running and take advantage of the steam. Now, we don't want your wife to think you're crazy or on some kind of a weird "steam" high, so explain to her that she could use a bit of humidity for her hair—and skin—too. Or have a good long shower—the longer the better, especially if you have willing company.

During all my travels I've gotten to know many pilots and flight attendants (who used to be called stewards and stewardesses), and all of them complain that the hours spent in pressurized cabins with no humidity makes their hair and skin dry and brittle, a complaint shared by doctors and nurses who work for hours every day in temperature-controlled operating or recovery rooms.

Saunas—A Mixed Blessing

While we're speaking about artificial heat, we should talk about the reputedly beneficial saunas which seem to be cropping up everywhere. Sweating off some of those pounds may seem like a good idea, but this approach is disastrous to your hair. A true sauna treatment features temperatures over 180 degrees F. (82.2 degrees C.), and hair can stand temperatures only up to 108 degrees F. (42.2 degrees C.). If you are a sauna aficionado, before you enter that hotbox, wet a Turkish towel in cold water and wrap it around your head in turban fashion.

While your body is being assaulted on all sides by that very intense heat, at least your hair will be moisturized. Also, when the cold wet turban becomes hot to your touch you'll know you've had enough and should get out of there. Because if you don't watch what you're doing with saunas, not only could you ruin your hair, but also, you could die from a heart attack. So, when you feel uncomfortable, leave the sauna room for a few minutes, rewet the towel turban with very cold water and then you can go back for a few more minutes if you're really a glutton for punishment. The important thing is that such intense heat should be kept away from direct contact with your hair.

Summer Stress

What you should do to protect your hair and head from the heat of summer can be expressed very simply in two words: cover it—with a white hat or cap. It's no accident that sailors, seamen and people working in the tropics have worn white or light-colored caps or hats or head coverings for thousands of years. White is the only color that deflects the ultraviolet rays of the sun—devastating for both hair and skin. But a white hat or cap also makes you feel cooler, since the hot sun bounces off it, as opposed to dark colors, which absorb the heat. Why do you think Queen Elizabeth's guards have been known to faint during the summer? Think of their hairy black hats. But in spite of the tropical climate, Jamaican guards don't faint because, sensibly, they are wearing white hats.

While this rule about hats is easy to follow for trips to the beach or a pool, I'm always amazed that the most careful people (men and women alike) will go sightseeing or shopping the very next day without a protective hat, cap (or, for women, a smartly tied scarf). The same sun shines over the pool, the ocean and the ruins of Pompeii—and if you're hatless it can do the same amount of damage.

If a light-haired man is walking next to a dark-haired man, the Robert Redford type won't seem as uncomfortable in the sun because his blond hair naturally deflects the sun's rays. The Dustin Hoffman type will feel hot and ill at ease and will run for cover or put on a hat first. Ironically, Redford's hair will suffer more abuse because he doesn't feel the heat as much. In the long run, both men are better off if they wear a hat.

Swimming—Water Can Be Dangerous

Swimming in either salt water or chlorinated pools would pose no problems to the hair if everyone wore a bathing cap. Most people—male or female—who aren't Olympic swimmers refuse to wear them, so that's that.

But what your hair really needs to protect it from the salt or the chlorine is some kind of shield. Of course, you could coat it with vaseline or axle grease, but you wouldn't enjoy wearing this, and if you were swimming in a pool, your host or the country club wouldn't welcome you back. (And such heavy coatings of grease are difficult to remove afterward.) So, more realistically, take care of your hair when you're swimming via the following methods:

Beat Chlorine

A recent study showed that drinking chlorine-laced water can be dangerous for your health. On the other hand, without the purifying benefits of chlorine, you could get dysentery, typhoid or any number of other hazardous diseases. The point is, if drinking chlorinated water (which is diluted to a far greater extent than in any swimming pool) is harmful internally, it's easy to realize how treating your hair to a chlorine bath can be harmful externally.

I always tell my female clients to walk around the pool, showing off their gorgeous hair for five or ten minutes, and then work in undiluted cream rinse before diving in. I suggest you skip the first part of the formula for defying chlorine. As to the second part, if you think rubbing in some cream rinse is too effete, let me ask you a question. Do you think putting suntan oil or lotion on is less than macho? Of course you don't, especially if you have a lovely lady doing the application. So what's the difference? Is there a special taboo against protecting your hair although it's okay to protect your skin? I don't think so—and because I take care of my hair, I still have most of it.

Applying cream rinse is no big deal. Just pour a dollop into your hands and rub it through your hair. Then take the plunge.

The chlorine will be happy because it enjoys eating the cream rinse instead of your hair; your hair will be happy because it's protected from the chemicals; and the pool owner will be happy because if enough swimmers wearing cream rinses use the pool, the water will be softer than gallons of Downy could ever make it. And I will be happy because you're not destroying your hair that we're working so hard to improve. So, everybody's happy.

When you're through swimming, rinse your hair off with plain water; you don't have to take a shower, just put your head under one of the garden hoses all pool owners have in abundance. If you're at a public pool you can use the shower on the way out.

Fight Salt

During the winter, when you want to get your car out of the driveway, or make sure the mailman doesn't fall on the steps, you sprinkle these surfaces with salt or a salt compound. The ice melts, so nobody sues you for damages; but the driveway and the steps also show the damages of salt—pitting and scarring that gets worse over the years. In a much diminished way—but the same process, nonetheless—this is what salt water does to your hair. I love salt water, and my favorite vacations are those spent near the sea. And salt water in small doses can be good for your scalp (not your hair) and good therapy for your body, but continued exposure to salt water can make your hair dry and brittle. While you apply a cream rinse before swimming in a chlorinated pool, before plunging into the surf you should coat your hair with conditioner.

And then, after your swim, rinse off, as usual, with plain, "sweet" water treatment.

Get Some Help from Your Barber or Stylist

In addition to the help you give your hair by appropriate seasonal care, your barber or stylist can help you too by applying special treatments.

There are treatments and there are treatments. First of all, you have to know what they can and can't do for you; all treatments are corrective only within the limits of cosmetology. If your problem is not simply external or cosmetic, if your hair is suffering because of an illness, or stress, or a vitamin deficiency, the treatments may help, but they will not cure your condition. In such cases an honest and expert' barber, stylist or "unisex" hairdresser will recommend that you see your regular doctor or, better yet, a dermatologist or trichologist.

Aside from these medically or psychologically caused problems, everyone with normal hair should have a professional protein-based heat treatment in the spring and in the fall. If your hair is very damaged or has been abused, then I recommend such a treatment every three months.

With all the advances in modern technology, there has been a corresponding increase in the number of therapeutic salon treatments which can be offered. Some have been described by manufacturers as being effective in ten minutes' time or twenty minutes' time. Some do not require heat as part of the treatment processing. I feel, however, that an ideal protein treatment, which acts as a filler for depleted hair, requires an hour's time: twenty minutes to "open" the hair shingle, twenty minutes to deposit the treatment into the hair and twenty minutes to close it again.

The word *filler* is crucial here. I can only explain it to you by describing a slab of wood that's been tied to the back bumper of your car and dragged around while you drive through town for a week or so. At the end of that time, aside from the state of your nerves, the state of that piece of wood will be very antiqued, to say the least. It will be pitted, stained, scarred. And that is actually what your hair looks like before a revitalizing protein treatment.

There are several good protein-based treatments available to professionals.

Can You Do It Yourself?

Frequently, on radio or TV shows I share a panel with a famous movie or television star who usually wants to hear my opinions about her fabulous homemade remedies for fantastic hair. I listen politely while she says, "I always use mayonnaise on my hair," but I ache to tell this well-known beauty that she would benefit more by *eating* that mayonnaise. Most commercial products (and we do have a wonderful variety in this country) are better and less expensive to use than "granny's goodies." The one home remedy I could recommend for hair conditioning is using oil, and this has been successfully employed by clever people for thousands of years. Although the oil particles are really too large to penetrate the cuticle (see Chapter Seven), to some degree they can lubricate the hair. It's an easy recipe. Simply heat about half a cup of sunflower-seed oil, olive oil, or any other vegetable oil you have on hand in a Pyrex cup or a small saucepan, and apply it all over your hair and scalp. Then wrap your head in a damp, hot towel and sit for a few minutes under a hair dryer. Rinse out—you may have to shampoo your hair three times to get out all the excess oil—and there you are. Your hair will be shinier and less flyaway after this type of treatment.

There are commercial conditioners you can use at home between professional treatments that you might like to try instead.

I think, though, at this point, I have to say, that whether you use commercial products, or mayonnaise, or olive oil to condition your hair, it's most important to reemphasize what we said at the beginning: modern life takes a great deal out of our hair and if you want it to behave well and look well, it's worth making an effort to put back what you've taken out.

Chapter Four

Face It—All About Hairstyles and Cuts

Somebody once said, "There's nothing new under the sun," and although with modern technology, space trips and the like, I have to disagree with a total generalization, when it comes to hairstyling, the adage is probably on target. Crew cuts aren't new: Alexander the Great invented them a few thousand years ago. Beards and mustaches and long hair aren't new: they were popular in pre-Roman times, during the Middle Ages and all through the nineteenth century.

The best thing about hairstyles for men today is that most things "go": choose whichever style you want, and within that framework, most men will avoid the extremes—ponytails or military crew cuts. The best style for a man is always a classic cut that takes into consideration his facial structure as well as his hair type. While some variations can be made in terms of current fashions—a little longer or shorter at the neck or sideburns, a little fuller at the front or back, a higher or lower part, or no part—a man should learn which haircut or style suits him best and stay with it.

Proportion

This is the key in choosing a hairstyle. You never want your face to look too small or too large for your body. The face is only one-sixth of the head and one forty-second of the body. Men should learn to look at all sides of their heads, not just their faces, for correct proportions. Unfortunately, most men look in the mirror and see just their heads, like John the Baptist's head on a plate.

But when you look at other people, you look from head to toe—and other people look at you from head to toe, not just from your head up. When I went to a military academy as a boy, there was a sign near the exit of our dormitory:

> Look at your head
> Look at your helmet
> Look at your collar
> Look at your jacket
> Look at your trousers
> Look at your shoes
> Now you may go out.

Total Concept

Aside from proportions, your hair must reflect your entire look as a man, as a person. If you spend your life working outdoors as an engineer, wearing rugged tweeds and boots, a short, businesslike cut might not be right for the image; it might seem in conflict with your life-style. On the other hand, if you're a stockbroker, given to three-piece suits, hair that's too long, or a Kris Kristofferson beard might offset the image and respect you're trying to establish. The best example of harmony in total concept I can think of is President Reagan, who never looks as if he just had a haircut, looks perfect, on target, always. This should be every man's goal.

Part of establishing the total concept about your appearance depends on outside influences, too. Maybe you like to influence the way your lady looks. You like long hair, and she tries to please you. Or, you like blond, short hair, and she tries to please you by cutting and then bleaching her once long and chestnut-colored locks. But just as she should not adopt any drastic look for your sake (I would try to dissuade any customer from cutting long hair short and bleaching dark hair blond because her boyfriend liked it that way), you shouldn't take on her influences either, unless you agree they are right for you. After all, it works both ways.

If your woman is crazy about the shaven Yul Brynner or Telly Savalas no-hair style, perhaps she should be with either of these men, instead of you. Shaving your head, or bleaching it, or permanenting it into an afro should not be considered lightly. These are major steps that take a long time to live with . . . and a long time to grow out of.

However, hair does grow, so now and then you can afford to indulge a whim (yours or hers)—a beard, a mustache, a longer or shorter style—but the major point always is to aim at being true to what will look best on you. One friend of mine was crazy about a movie actor who had a thick, luxuriant mustache; it gave him a real look of strength, and she worshiped him from afar, as the saying goes. Then, a few months ago, in another film, he had shaved off the mustache and suddenly he looked weak, vulnerable and not so special at all. My friend quickly fell out of love with her dream man. Really, that actor should have stayed with his brush.

Fine, Thick, Curly, Scrubby

Selecting hairstyles and total concepts are fine—except that you always have to consider the type of hair you have in relation to the look you want to achieve. Men have come to this realization only lately, although women have reckoned with the beast for years. Until recently, men, like an army of well-trained robots, would dutifully walk into their barbershop once a month or so, sit in a chair, put themselves into the hands of their barbers, whom they asked only to "take a little off where it's needed," close their eyes, and awaken to a haircut that was perhaps too short but definitely looked exactly like every other man's haircut.

Now, men are learning that their hair may not be right for a certain look, and they definitely do not want to look like every other man. You can't adopt a Paul Newman, short, tight, curly hairstyle if you have fine, limp hair. You'll never achieve Donald Sutherland's laid-back, classic, fair-haired look if your hair is thick, dark and wiry. Burt Reynolds can't make his hair look like the late William Holden's (and why should he?), and Prince Charles can't make his hair look like Robert De Niro's (and why should he?).

Part of the Question

Whether or not to part your hair and, if so, on which side to part it also figures in any decisions about styling. Now, some men find it easy to decide where to place a part—and it goes smack in the middle. Rudolph Valentino pulled off this look with great panache, and so does John Travolta half a century later. But the major reason they can is that they both were or are extremely handsome men and therefore, almost anything they did or do will work.

For the rest of us, this isn't the case. Every face has two different sides: an angelic side and a diabolic side. (Look at yourself in profile from both the left and the right side and you'll realize each side is just a little different.) Unfortunately, the diabolic or less attractive side always wins the center-part battle, not your more appealing side. A middle part, therefore, is esthetically hazardous because in addition to pointing up the dark side of you, it also plays up your worst features—a bumpy nose, a disappearing upper lip, a receding chin line. This type of hairstyle should only be worn by two types of men: the very ugly (for whom there is little hope anyway) or, as mentioned above, the very handsome who can get away with anything.

The 99 percent of men who are left should decide on a style with no part or a side part. In the latter case, the question is which side. Before you protest that this couldn't possibly matter, listen to some scientific details that make a case for the right side. Most of us sleep on the right side of the face during most of the night. (Even scientists can't explain why, but this is a fact established after two years of research in Germany.) Since we spend so much time sleeping on the right the hair on the right side of the head tends to be thinner and finer on everybody than the hair on the left side. (You'll find less hair on your right eyebrow than on your left, too, as an instant indicator that what I'm saying is accurate.)

In addition, although hair follicles grow all around the base of the head in a uniform circle, on top of the head the follicles grow from the left to the right. If you have very thick hair, this may not make much of a difference, but if you need all the help you can get—and a few more centimeters of height, too—part your hair on the right, *against* the growth, for natural body. A right-side part has your hair doing push-ups for you and you are automatically exercising your scalp by parting it on this side.

One more point: it may seem more natural for you to part your hair on the left, but remember that when you make that part you're looking in a mirror, which gives you a reverse image. You may spend only two or three minutes a day combing or styling your hair (and that's all the time you should spend gazing into a mirror unless you're a total narcissist or a well-paid actor or model), but the rest of the world sees you for twenty-three hours and fifty-seven minutes (minus the time you spend asleep) and they see not only your head but your total image, as we've said.

If you wear your hair parted, try it on the right for a few days and you'll see that I'm right. (You may remember that our ex-President, Jimmy Carter, made just such a part change early in his incumbency, and it definitely improved his appearance.)

Special Circumstances

Your age, occupation, even your life-style, count, too. While a college student can wear a natural or afro style, this might not suit the image of a forty-five-year-old tax lawyer who wants to look dignified. However, a sportsman or a man who spends a great deal of his time outdoors might find the natural type of cut perfectly suited to his way of life—if he has the right hair for this style. And life-styles and hairstyles also change—and should change as a reflection of personal fluctuations. I remember when H. R. Haldeman, Nixon's right-hand man, favored a crew cut, which made him look very authoritarian—perfect for his job. After he left the White House staff in the Watergate flood, it's interesting that he adopted a softer-looking style which made him appear less rigid.

Speaking Personally

I have two rules that I'd like to suggest, and feel free to break them if you like, but they've worked for me and most of the men whose hair I've cared for over the years.

The first is, if you think a natural afro style is your best bet, make sure you can match it with a young-looking, wrinkle-free face—because afros and wrinkles don't work, whether you're a man or a woman of a certain age.

Think of a mirror. When you cut your hair very short, and you combine this with nature's normal lines around the eyes and mouth, and then you "electrify" the hair with tight waves, the effect is really like that of shattering the serenity of a mirror by hitting it with a rock. Everything is jagged and sharp; instead of smooth planes which erase age, you have a conglomeration of harsh angles which play up the worst time-telling accents: wrinkles upon wrinkles. I firmly believe older men should have slightly longer hair, straighter hair, which will take emphasis away from those facial lines and achieve a more serene look.

My second rule is that it's a mistake for men to have their hair cut very short on the front of the head. This is where hair loss always occurs first and to the greatest degree. By keeping the hair longer in front, not only will you strengthen the roots, which will make them more resistant to fallout, but you'll also be avoiding the tendency of hair to shed through a natural equalization process.

When hair is cut all one length, it is in harmony with the way nature meant it to grow. Try this "laboratory" test yourself if you want to prove the facts about uneven hair lengths. Take a small mammal that doesn't shed, such as a poodle dog, and shave one leg. Within two or three weeks he will begin to drop the hair on the other leg in nature's way of equalizing the situation. Although I haven't had to resort to giving dogs experimental haircuts, in my salon I've seen hundreds of instances of this equalization in women who have had bangs or layered haircuts and then had to suffer through problems with the rest of the hair.

So, when you see a balding man who has very long hair in front, you shouldn't laugh at him for making obvious efforts to camouflage the balding. In fact, he's really making a sensible effort to hold on to his hair.

The best example I can give you is my own case history. When I was a young man in the navy, like every other recruit I had to have a crew cut and my hair immediately succumbed to shock. Almost over-

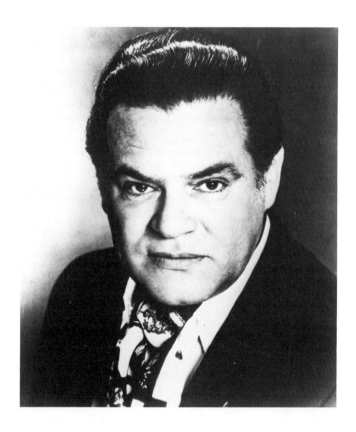

night it seemed thinner. As soon as I became an officer and was allowed to wear it longer, I began to grow the front section, and ever since then I've always kept it six inches long in front. Now I don't look like an overage beatnik because the front is brushed back, I keep the sideburns trimmed and I wear the back fairly short—and I will probably never be bald!

Here are some current, classic styling ideas I recommend from stylists in the United States and abroad whose work has been collected by Pivot Point International, a worldwide training and information source for hair stylists and designers.

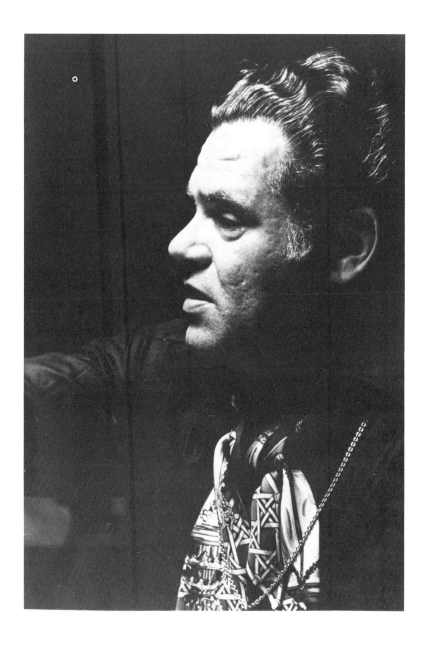

Manhattan

Designed by Thomas Esrey for Pivot Point International, this is an excellent look for the man who prefers longer hair but whose profession demands an always impeccable and well-groomed appearance. The cut can be varied to be worn straight back and off the face or with a side-part variation. The lines of the cut point out good masculine features and create a no-nonsense frame for the face. Because the hair is styled to look full, a side benefit of Manhattan is a vigorous and youthful look that works well with fine to medium hair.

As an example of the difference in appearance the right haircut and style can achieve, compare these "before" and "after" pictures.

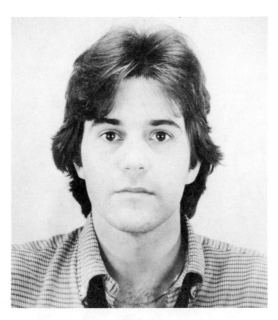

Before

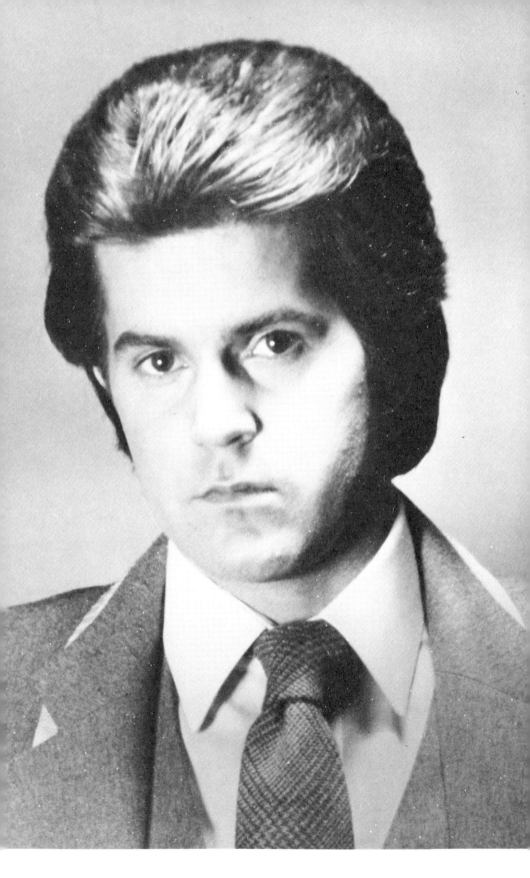

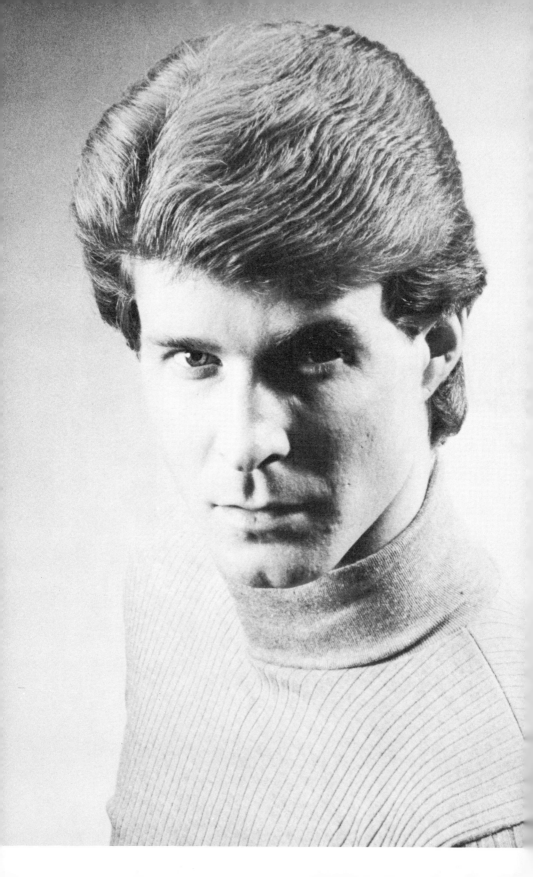

Beau

As stated often in this book, one of the major problems is dealing with fine hair, which tends to become limp and look out of control. An excellent solution to this problem is provided by Howard Alberts with his Beau design, which uses all-over one-length layering to achieve a crisp, clean look that requires minimum care.

The Beau design emphasizes an overall square form cut following the natural growth directions, with straight angles which minimize the length of the model's face while emphasizing his best features.

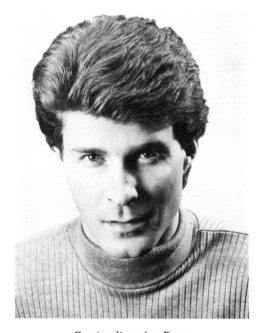

Cutting lines for Beau

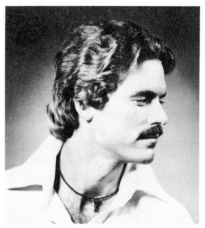

Before

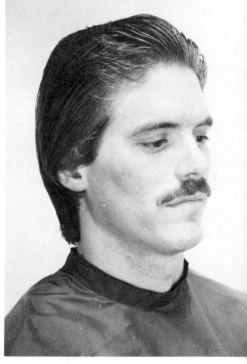

Version 1

Casino

This versatile design was created by master stylist Jean-Pierre DeMarquet of Paris and is a good example of an ideal hairstyle—clean-cut, trim and flexible enough to meet quick changes in life-style from business to sports, as illustrated by these photographs.

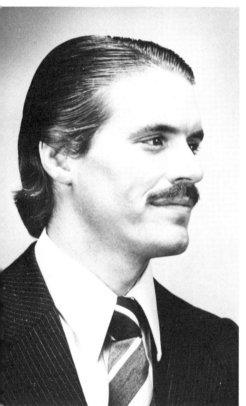

Version 2

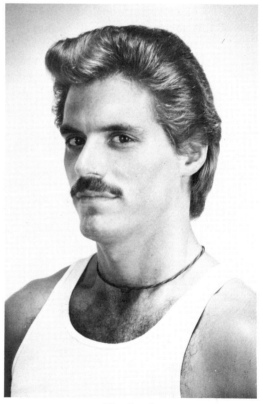

Version 3

Maestro

An excellent example of the importance of facial and hair analysis before deciding on a hairstyle is provided in this design, Maestro, by Pierre Zanca of Spain. The model's hair-growth pattern, hair texture and bone structure were first considered to determine balance and proportion. The result was a sculptured design created by following a square form through the top and sides. The back was layered in order to take advantage of existing wave texture rather than fighting the wave. Instead of the straggly, distracting appearance of the model before the Maestro styling, we now have a precise and carefully balanced design that is appropriate as well as flattering for a mature professional man.

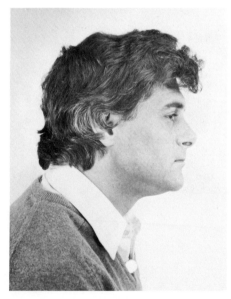

Before

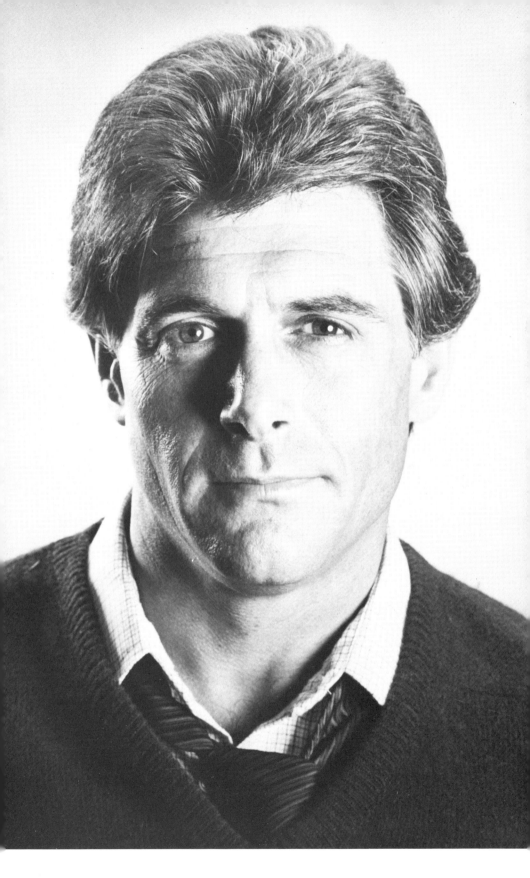

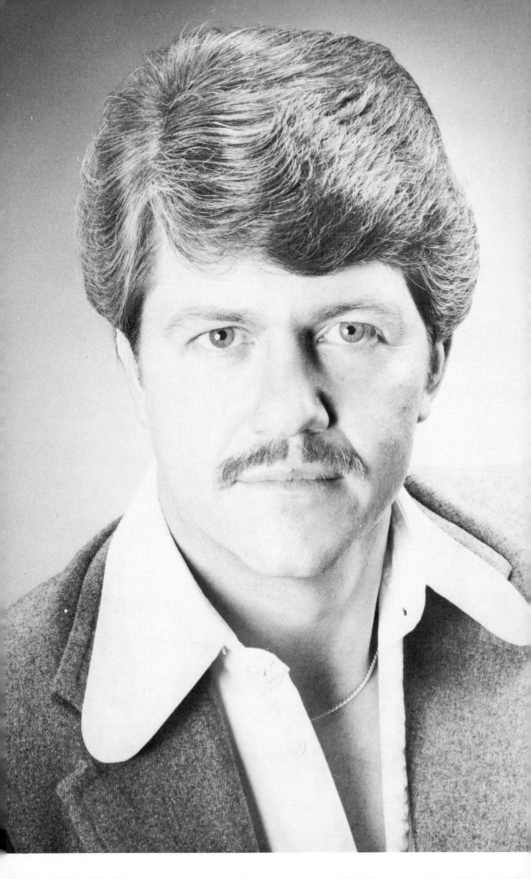

Baccarat

An excellent example of how thick, wavy hair can be tamed for results that not only enhance the appearance but also are more suitable for image and life-style is shown in this design, Baccarat, engineered by Franklin of London, England.

This man, in his forties, was proud of his thick, full head of hair, but what looked okay on the beach looked erratic in his office, as illustrated by the "before" photograph.

Franklin removed the bulk at the nape of the neck and sides, cut the hair in a square form which flatters the man's face and goes with the wave and not against it and styled the hair forward with a side part to give a more businesslike look. In line with my emphasis on total concept, the model's mustache was also trimmed in order to "clean up" his complete facial image.

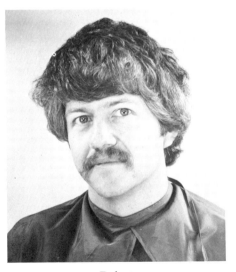

Before

Uptown

This is another example of an urbane look that's right for big city living, designed by Dennis Mattos of Crystal Lake (Illinois). Unfussy and unflappable, this style transforms formerly dry and thin-looking hair into an easy-to-manage style. As indicated by the "before" picture, the model looked unsophisticated and undistinguished. After the design, not only does the artful cut give the illusion of more body and hair, but the resulting style gives the model a definite look of savoir faire and distinction.

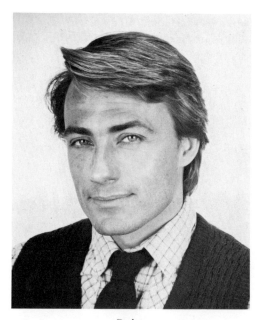

Before

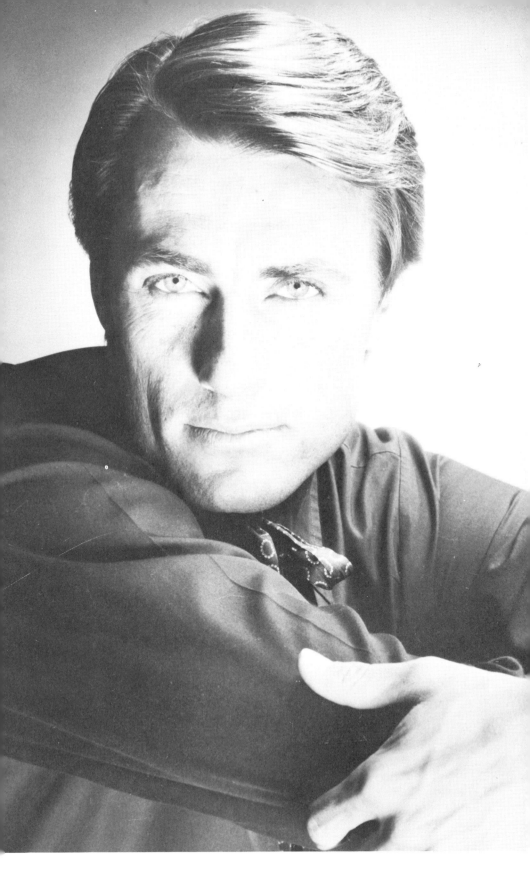

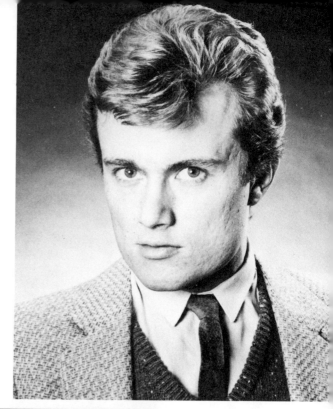

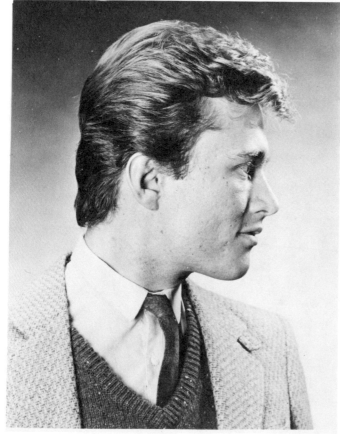

Varsity

Here, Pierre Zanca turns his styling innovations toward the needs of a younger man who also wants a polished image. The design is very youth-ful-looking, as suits the model's age, and the shorter, layered cut is very practical and easy to care for. Varsity is an excellent example of how a hair design based on hair texture and type (in this case, fine with a slight wave) when combined with facial structure can really change one's total appearance, as indicated by the "before" and "after" pictures.

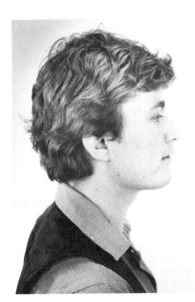
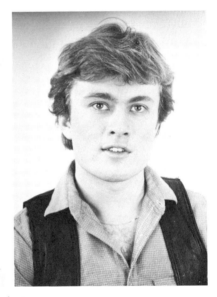

Before

Teenage Hairstyle

The universal rule for teenage haircuts is that they must be extremely easy to care for. Teenage boys, unlike teenage girls, don't want to spend more than a few minutes a day worrying about their hair. And they want to see a stylist as infrequently as possible, perhaps in youthful rebellion against a mother's frequent plea: "Won't you *please* get a haircut?"

Not only are the two examples we've included easy to maintain, but the result in both cases is a definite improvement in appearance.

This young man's hair was totally out of shape and the long bangs and hair below the collar line made his face look longer and emphasized his small jaw. His hair is very fine and required layered shaping to maintain line and literally fall into place. As indicated by the "after" photograph, the new style shortens the length of his face and emphasizes his eyes rather than his jaw and mouth.

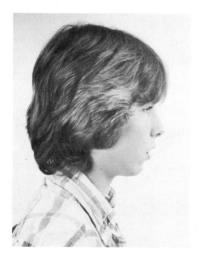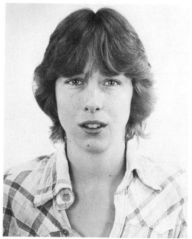

Before

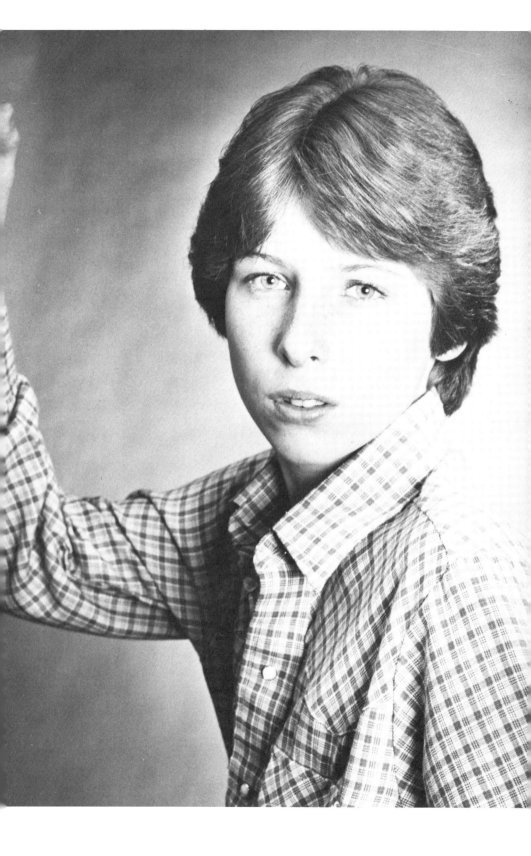

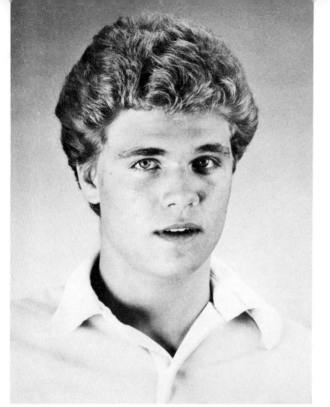

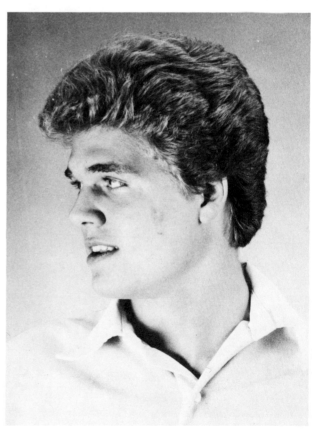

Teenage Hairstyle

There is no question that this college student would be considered handsome even with hair down to his shoulders—or possibly with no hair at all. But even the very good-looking can benefit from an improved hairstyle. This young man has very wiry, dry hair, with too much bulk in the front and at the sides, which creates an unkempt look and actually calls attention to a rigid, too-square jaw. Once the bulk was removed and the hair lifted off the face at the forehead, his face looked longer, the jaw was less dominant and his best features, the eyes and eyebrows, took over control.

This student had abused his hair via swimming and too much exposure to the sun, so among the recommendations made when his hair was restyled was the use of cream conditioners and the practice of frequent massage to encourage circulation.

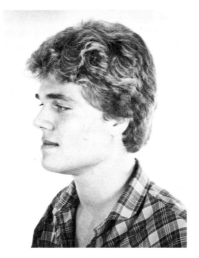

Before

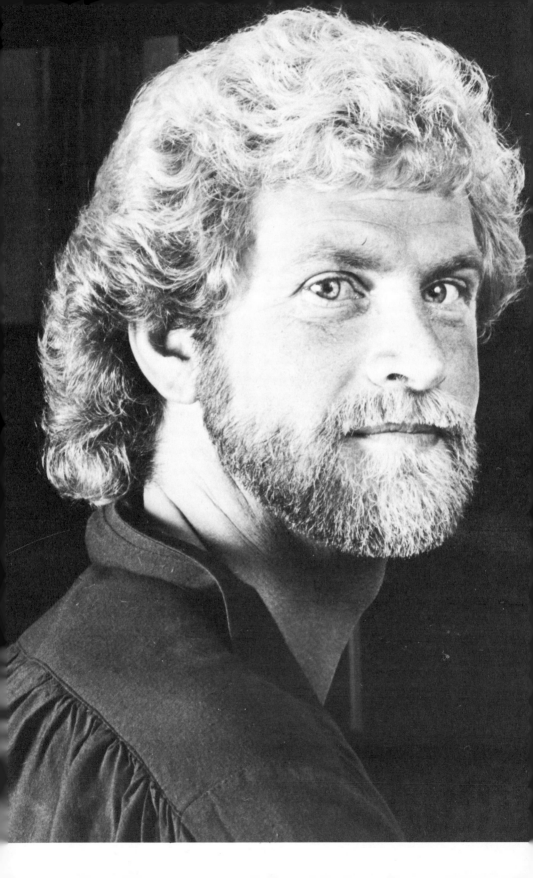

Commodore

In this design, the sportsman, whose hair was restyled by Karel van de Tonnekreek of Holland, had a lot of good things going for him: a very rugged look, abundant, sun-bleached hair and good facial features. But he wanted a neater look, and felt his hair looked skimpy on top and at the base of his head. And it did. Karel van de Tonnekreek removed bulk and extra length, gave the model a body permanent for height and substance on top, sides and crown, and reshaped his mustache; his beard needed only a trim.

The difference illustrated by the "before" and "after" pictures is a classic example of how the right haircut and styling (which in this case included a body permanent) can make even the best-looking man look better!

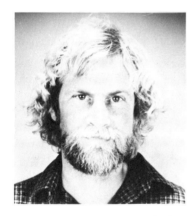
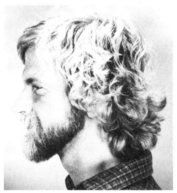

Before

Mustaches and Beards

In several of the hair designs illustrated above, it's evident that a mustache and/or a beard contribute to the total look and have to be styled accordingly: neither a mustache nor a beard should be allowed to grow helter-skelter, with its owner hoping for the best.

Following are diagrams of mustaches on their own, beards on their own and combinations of the two. If you currently grow a mustache and/or a beard, or are thinking of adopting either or both facial hairstyles, use these diagrams as guides to what suits your face, your total concept and the hair you have to work with. It might be worthwhile to have several Xerox copies made of a facial blowup, and use a pencil to doodle in various mustaches and/or beards.

While you're doodling, keep these points in mind:

Mouth-Magnifying Mustaches

The mustache expresses a man's essential character because it either magnifies a strong mouth or camouflages a weak one. A mustache can tell the world that a man is meticulous and orderly, casual and free-wheeling, debonair and sophisticated, swashbuckling (to use that unfashionable but apt word) and rugged. But there are some combinations that don't work well at all. A down-turned mustache teamed with droopy eyes will give you a hangdog expression. A small mustache perched under a prominent nose will produce a slightly comic look. Everything must be in balance. Remember, too, that a mustache, when well designed, can reshape an unbalanced mouth and conceal less-than-perfect teeth.

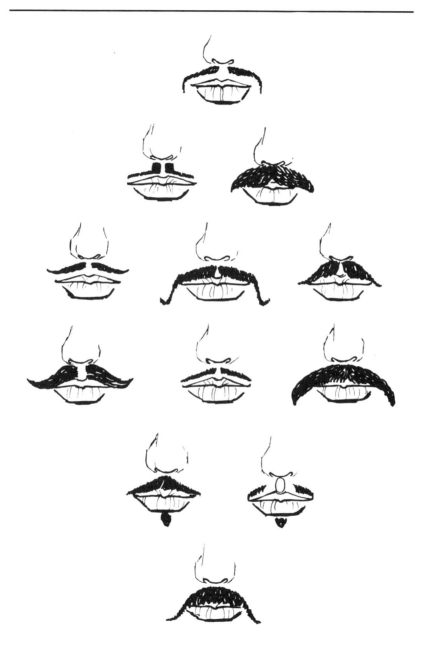

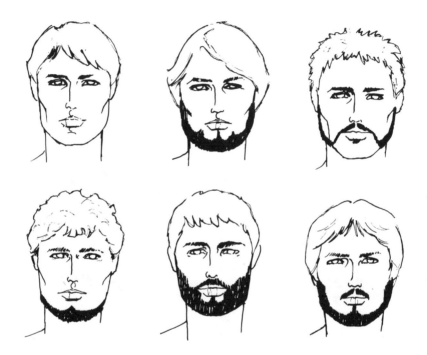

Face-Framing Beards

A beard represents a fashion statement more and more men are making these days, but the beard of the eighties is a far cry from the wild, anything-goes beard of the sixties. The contemporary beard is sculpted to fit the face *and* the hairstyle *and* the personality of its owner. A beard can open up the face to give a frank, masculine look, strengthen a jawline, highlight strong cheekbones, make a man look more sophisticated, or more dashing, or more romantic, all depending on the style chosen, in combination with the face and the hair texture and cut.

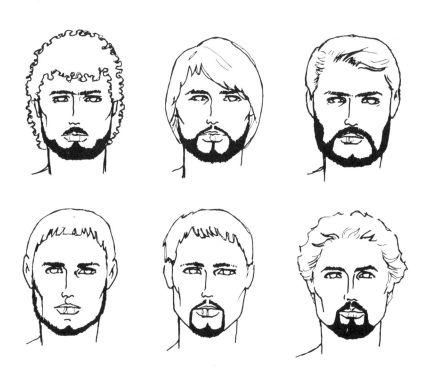

PART TWO

Looking Good –
More's at Stake than
a Haircut

Chapter Five

Shape Up— What to Use and How to Care for Your Hair Day by Day

At no other time in history have there been so many products and kinds of equipment and special treatments and processes to improve the way your hair grows, looks, feels, thrives, behaves. In 1964, a total of $1,066,810,000 was spent on hair care products in the United States. Fifteen years later, the figure had more than doubled. There have been many excellent developments, but there are also some distinctly bad products and practices which many men (and women, too) adopt because of confusion or lack of knowledge.

Of course, a good professional who understands hair, who knows more about hair than simply styling it or cutting it, will try to educate you and set you on the right track to caring for your hair yourself between visits to his salon. Unfortunately, many stylists have a superficial background in what really makes hair tick, and it's up to you to be the master of your fate when it comes to your hair. This book gives you the information you need; the goal is that your hair should look as well every day as it does when you leave the barber. Taking care of your hair should be a joy, not a chore.

You can't, however, do a crash program in one day to break the habits or change the results of years of improper care, just as you can't lose fifty pounds in a day or build muscles in one day. You will have to be patient for six months to a year until all the cumulative results we've been explaining take hold.

Start with the Right Comb and Brush

As I said earlier, the best brush for anybody—man, woman or child—is always one made out of natural bristles, because hair is hair and natural bristle is also hair. You will not have friction between different substances. There are different brushes for different lengths of hair, but since most men have hair no longer than six inches, the choice should be a "club" brush, a flat brush which can be used in a flat motion all around the head without rotating the wrist. While I don't usually recommend expensive products, I will always suggest buying a good hairbrush; it's an investment that will last for ten to twenty years and if you amortize the price in this way, the cost is well worth it.

Whichever brush you choose, always remember: *never* brush your hair when it's wet, because this is the time when hair is most elastic and will stretch, and the stretching ultimately can snap the hair. Instead, use a wide-toothed comb or let the hair dry naturally until you're ready to style it.

Natural products are also the best material for combs, but unfortunately, when combs were made of ram's horn or bull's horn or tortoiseshell, if dropped on a hard floor, the comb would splinter and the effect would be like using a razor blade to comb your hair. Today, we still use (and I personally prefer) tortoiseshell combs, but now they are bound with plastic and cellulose, and if they are dropped, they are so solid and safe that no splitting of the hair occurs because of broken or abraded teeth. Kent of London manufactures my line of combs; I recommend the George Michael Comb ✗90, with coarse teeth, for thick or wiry hair, and the George Michael Comb ¥100, with fine teeth, for fine or thin hair.

A word here about using a comb: there's nothing virile about raking it through your hair as if you were raking up last year's leaves. I've seen people comb their dog's hair more kindly than they comb their own.

Take Care of Your Tools

In the same way that you keep your hair clean, you have to keep your tools clean, and while I'm never one to denigrate parents, most mothers and fathers I know never taught their little boys (or their little girls) this primary rule. Yet could anything be more elementary? Would you use a dirty rag to polish the car you've just washed?

At least once a month, fill a basin or your sink with mild suds (or use shampoo as the sudsing agent) and give your combs and brush a bath. Don't let the brush soak for any length of time (just enough to clean the bristles) and then rinse carefully with cold water, shake it, place on its side for half an hour and allow the brush to dry face up. To clean your combs, use an old toothbrush to get between the teeth and then dry with a terry towel.

Turn On the Current—Dryers, Blowers, Styling Sticks, et al.

Generally, I'm against anything that involves applying very hot heat to the hair and scalp, whether that heat comes from the sun, a sauna or an electric appliance. As you know by now, hair is strong but fragile, and heat is one of its worst enemies. After shampooing, my preference is either to towel-dry the hair (which provides a healthy massage) or to comb through it gently and let it dry naturally.

However, with some styles and some types of hair, a blowdryer is necessary to achieve the final result. If this is the case, keep a few precautions in mind: set the blowdryer or styling stick on warm to moderate temperature, *not* the hottest. This will probably be about 108 degrees F. and therefore not harmful, because 108 degrees represents your regular body heat of 98.6 plus 10 degrees, which is a natural habitat for the hair. Hotter than that, you hurt your hair and your scalp. The second precaution is to try to minimize the amount of time spent using an electric appliance. This is difficult at first if you're trying to get the hang of using a blowdryer or re-create a new style so it looks the way it looked in the hands of your stylist, but in time you should be able to accomplish your grooming in about five minutes. If it takes more than that, you don't have a good cut, or you don't have the right cut for your hair.

Put On a Coat—Sprays, Thickeners

Products that coat the hair are used for one of two purposes: to give it more body and to make it stay the way it looks right after styling. You can achieve body by rinsing your hair with cold water after shampooing, but this may not be enough. So, you turn to any of the hair thickeners on the market. These work by coating hair strands with a liquid that provides more bulk. That's not bad. The only problem is that the bulk is a little sticky to the hand, now, and if you're mated to a lady, or hoping to connect with one, who likes to run her fingers through your hair, the going becomes a little tacky, in the true sense of the word (like glue). (My new body builder, Instar, has been developed to work with minimal application to avoid this buildup.)

The same objection might be raised with hair sprays; but in addition, these can make your hair look pasted into place, and any kind of buildup is suffocating to the scalp. A little judicious use of spray is okay, though. Most men comb their hair once or twice a day—unless caught in a windstorm or participating in a heavy game of tennis—so if you know that your hair is going to stay pretty much in place, you can go about other business, important business, without worrying about whether or not you look as if you just got out of bed.

The key word is judicious. Never put layer upon layer of thickener or spray on your hair (shampoo more often to counteract this), and don't fall into that old trap of if a little helps, a little more will help a lot more. I don't like stiff-looking hair on women, but it's equally unattractive on men!

Special Problems—Problem Hair

You follow all the suggestions and they don't quite work. Why? Because your hair is fine or coarse, thick or thin, frizzy or dry. Here are some points to keep in mind when caring for it or having it styled:

Dry Hair

It's crying for oil, don't deny it—just as you wouldn't let your car run when you know the dip-stick calls for a quart or more. Feed your hair with Wildroot Cream Oil (don't raise your eyebrows until you try it for a few weeks). First use a couple of drops and see how that works to determine how much is enough. Then increase or decrease accordingly, because you don't want to look like Greaseball Charlie. But the Wildroot will help, because dry hair is very flyaway and hard to manage.

Oily Hair

This hair is crying out for shampoo; wash more often, using a cream shampoo, and make an extra effort to wash your combs and brushes. If they aren't clean, you're just distributing more grease to compound the problem.

Fine Hair

You can't turn a sow's ear into a silk purse, and you can't turn fine hair into a luxuriant Dean Martin head if your hair is more like Luciano Pavarotti's (never mind the very great difference in voices; Dean has the hair and Luciano has the voice). Instead, fine hair should be worn longer and should be cut with a definite line.

Coarse Hair

Don't try to force this type of hair into trendy styles that call for engineering and line. Coarse hair goes where it wants to go, and your best hope for keeping it good-looking is to follow the path your hair wants to take. You can, however, calm coarse hair down a bit by faithful use of conditioners, as described earlier.

Frizzy Hair

This is weak hair, dry hair. First moisturize it with Wildroot or another oil-based product. Then let it grow a little, because longer hair is less frizzy. Or don't fight it at all, and wear your hair in a natural style. Despite the fact that it is already wavy, a body permanent may help give it more bulk and control.

Cowlicks

Wear your hair longer, because short hair makes a cowlick more prominent. Always comb your hair in the direction of the cowlick, not against it, or you'll look like some character in a comic strip—I think his name was Dennis the Menace. If you have two cowlicks, don't worry about it at all, because only geniuses have two cowlicks.

Hair and Sports

Exercise is good for the hair; sports are good for the mind and the body and therefore the hair. But engaging in sports takes a certain toll on the hair, which requires extra care and consideration. If you're a wrestler by trade or avocation, maybe it's better to be bald so that your opponent can't get a handhold. On the other hand, you might just be more vulnerable without hair because you have no built-in cushion to protect you from bumps and bruises.

Sports do put greater strains on your hair. Hockey players wear helmets and perspire, tennis players perform in the blazing sun usually without headgear, swimmers are in and out of chlorinated water constantly. In any of these cases, the hair loses, even though you win the match.

In hockey, or polo, or baseball, any sport where you're wearing a hat, you're going to perspire more, and the body gets rid of its poisons and sweat through the skin. Scalp is skin. After the game, it's not enough to shower and wet your hair; shampoo it, the same way you'd soap your underarms or other areas that do or don't have hair.

In cases where you are actively involved in a sport where you don't wear a hat, such as tennis or racquetball or jogging, after you've displayed your athletic prowess (while displaying your head for a couple of hours to the brutal sun), do yourself and your hair a favor by coddling it with a good rich cream conditioner—and follow this formula every time you expose your hair. If swimming is your sport, coat your hair with cream rinse before entering a pool, and afterward, always be sure to rinse your hair with fresh water.

Perhaps the sport I would recommend to most men is golf (although personally I'm not a golfer), because it's calmer, most golfers wear hats during play and ultimately it's a very relaxing interlude (even though one must concentrate fiercely). But the bottom line, really, is that the best sport is the one that turns you on the most— whether it's car racing or playing volleyball. Keep in mind, though, that your favorite sport may play havoc with your hair.

The important point is to be aware of stresses and strains on your hair, as well as your total physical being. It's not enough to be concerned about your hair: you must also keep everything in balance. Some men go to hair specialists or dermatologists or trichologists for treatments, massages, pomades, injections, even transplants. With all that, if you overuse a blowdryer afterward, you rob yourself of anything good the specialists have suggested or tried. It's true that some people have very healthy heads and can use a blowdryer twenty-six hours a day—but that is probably not the case with you.

I have a good friend who is a captain on a neighboring yacht in my marina. His hair is thinning on top in a pattern that is not natural, not caused by hereditary balding. J. has spent a great deal of money and time with specialists, but nobody told him not to sit on the aft deck in the sun during the hottest time of the day from ten in the morning until three in the afternoon. His hair is being destroyed by the ultraviolet rays of the sun. He is throwing his money and time away unless he learns to protect his head from these grueling rays. A good analogy is that his scalp is like a desert—and all you can grow in a desert is one or two cactus plants and that's it.

If you're not prepared to take care of your hair on a day-by-day basis, to follow the rules, all the specialists and special products in the world won't help you grow and maintain healthy hair.

Chapter Six

Change It—Hair Coloring, Bleaching, Straightening or Permanenting

I've seen a lot of changes in men's attitudes in the last few decades, and most of them I applaud heartily. In the move to liberate women, spearheaded mostly by women, one end result has been the liberation of men. Now a man is liberated (not tamed, mind you) to take on a lot of responsibilities as well as enjoy a great many more pleasures that formerly were considered "for women only."

Today he is liberated enough to enjoy cooking, caring for his children (much more active fathering than previously), and sharing in household chores without feeling he's doing "women's work." He's also more liberated and individualistic about himself and how he looks and what he wears. He knows that while the three-piece gray-flannel suit isn't the only uniform he should adopt, he doesn't have to prove he's with it by wearing jeans all the time either. He's interested in the total concept of masculinity and as part of that interest is into sports, exercise, foods, vitamins, physical fitness, even skin and hair care. It is a search for self-improvement, and this carries over into thinking about improving the look and behavior of hair by changing it—coloring or bleaching or permanenting or even straightening it, in addition to normal haircuts and styling changes.

But while I cheer the general move toward self-improvement, I have to put up a hand of caution when it comes to drastic changes for your hair. Let me tell you some of the pitfalls and other considerations, and then, armed with knowledge, you make your own decision.

Changing Natural Color

There are many instances where a change in hair color can mean a change in appearance and, in fact, a man's life-style and outlook. Some hair shades tend to fade out as one gets older; in other cases, prematurely gray hair may make a thirty-five-year-old man look as old as his father. So a little artificial help can mean a great deal in sprucing up an image. But right now I want to say very clearly that although coloring or bleaching or other techniques may improve appearance, I can't give such processes an unqualified green light.

To begin with, any permanent hair coloring changes the color and nature of the hair permanently. Just as you either are or are not a virgin, hair either is or is not virgin hair. And once it is colored or bleached, you are dealing with hair that will behave and react differently from that virgin hair you once owned.

Another reservation is the choice of color and type of hair-coloring technique used. Third, in recent years studies have been published showing a possible link between certain chemicals used in hair dyes and cancer. The major danger stems from the fact that these chemicals can be absorbed into the body through the skin and scalp. Consumers don't realize that the National Cancer Institute studies on which these fears were based utilized "maximum tolerated dose feeding," in which mice and rats were fed the maximum amount of test substances which they could tolerate—in this case the equivalent of a person *drinking* more than twenty-five bottles of hair dye a day for every day of his or her life.

Although new tests are under way, and some manufacturers have included warnings on their hair-coloring products as well as changed some of the formulations, I will always continue to be very conservative about applying hair-coloring solutions or other chemicals to the hair.

With these reservations clearly stated, here are the most common methods for changing your natural hair color:

Lightening or bleaching
Permanent tints
Frosting, streaking or highlighting
Semipermanent tints
Temporary rinses

Bleaches or Lighteners: What They Do to Your Hair

Whether they are called blonders, bleachers or highlighteners, all of these products do the same thing: they remove the color from your hair. When a bleaching product is applied, your hair can go through seven stages of color change:

Black
Brown
Red
Reddish gold
Gold
Yellow
Pale yellow or white

It's said, perhaps apocryphally, that Catherine de Medici, a very dynamic lady, first discovered the seven stages of bleaching while traveling from Italy to France to marry King Henry II. She stopped seven times, specifically to have her hair lightened gradually from darkest brown to palest blond, the hair color the French king most admired. Since Catherine is also credited with introducing haute cuisine to the then backward (at least in terms of food) French, we can only conclude that she was a very resourceful, clever woman. Think of her traveling to Paris not only with a retinue of cooks but also with a cadre of colorists!

Of course, the number of stages one goes through in bleaching is dictated not only by the original hair color but also by the shade desired. Often, bleaching alone will not produce the looked-for results. In these cases, after the single process of stripping color from the hair is done, a toner or tint must be added. This is known as *double-process bleaching.* I'm against double-process coloring for any amount of time because you first strip the natural oils from the scalp and hair (along with the color) and then you must hit your scalp and hair with harmful chemicals. As an analogy, the best toast with jam will always have a layer of butter applied to the bread before lavishing on the jam. This keeps the integrity of the bread; otherwise you would have a soggy mess. The same thing applies to double-process bleaching, which if practiced for any length of time will destroy the integrity of your hair and scalp.

On balance, if you were a towheaded youngster and now at thirty or forty or fifty find yourself with faded, nondescript brownish hair that makes you look tired, you might consider single-process bleaching. But keep in mind that the roots will have to be touched up once a month faithfully and the work must be done by a really experienced colorist. While a woman can possibly pull off an obviously bleached look, it is absolute anathema for a man to look like a "bleached blond" unless he belongs to a punk rock group.

There are also some types of mild lighteners that are used like shampoos, and several products even include a type of toner—but these achieve more of a sun-streaked look than a drastic change. Other bleaches use heat as an agent—either the sun or another heat-producing source, such as a hair dryer.

Permanent Hair Color

Today there are two kinds of permanent hair-coloring products available: *penetrating tints* and *coating tints*. Once they are applied, both types stay on the hair until it grows out or is changed by another process such as bleaching or color stripping. These tints don't wash out with shampoo and they can change the color of the hair completely, cover gray, darken, brighten or highlight.

Penetrating Tints

The most common permanent coloring technique used currently: The color penetrates the hair through the outer (cuticle) layer into the center layer (cortex), where the peroxide contained in the product oxidizes or develops into permanent pigment. This in turn is deposited into the hair shaft in the very same way natural pigment is deposited. The application of this tint, either with shampoo-in or cream formulas —deepens your natural (or existing) color to darker or richer shades, or can lighten it by several shades. The most lightening you can get with penetrating tints is four or five gradations of the same shade; to achieve any lighter effects the hair must be bleached.

The penetrating tints are the most desired form of permanent hair color because generally the natural-looking tones don't fade or turn off-color in time. The tinting action stops immediately when the hair is rinsed, so the color never turns darker. Beneficial conditioning oils are added to these formulas and as a result the texture of the hair improves. The chemicals contained in them are compatible with those included in permanent wave solutions. (Hair must always be colored after—*never before*—a permanent.)

Coating Tints

These products coat the outside (cuticle) layer of the hair with color and are seldom used today. Coating tints produce dull, flat, unnatural-looking shades because the coating principle prevents light from penetrating the cuticle so that natural highlights can be accentuated. As old-fashioned as this technique may be, however, it has come back into vogue recently with a craze for henna.

Now henna is so old that it came out of the Egyptian school of hairstyling some five thousand years ago. And it served a real purpose. Egyptians didn't like their hair because it was kinky. If you put something on your hair like shellac—in other words, a heavy coating—it will keep your hair straighter. Henna served the purpose but was very expensive: in terms of Egyptian currency it cost the equivalent of seventeen cows or so. Therefore, henna was used only by the very rich, which made it an immediate status symbol. Conveniently, the process had to be repeated only every six months. Not only did henna straighten the hair but it produced red shadings which the dark-haired Egyptians looked on as a sign of beauty.

Today, if hair is very porous, henna can impart not only reddish coloring but that shellaclike coating that gives better texture and shine to the hair. But if your hair is healthy and shiny, why use henna? And if you're trying to recapture reddish highlights of your long-ago youth, why use henna? Most important, henna is very difficult to remove once it's applied and the effect of the permanent coating makes giving any therapeutic treatments (such as a protein or other conditioning treatment) almost impossible.

Although henna is a natural product (made from a plant), which gives it a certain cachet these days, it has more disadvantages than advantages.

Highlighting—a.k.a. Frosting or Streaking

This is a vogue that's been around for the last decade or so, but only recently adopted as a trend for men. With highlighting (which in women's salons is also called frosting or streaking), individual strands of hair are permanently lightened. This can be effective for men with nondescript, dull brown hair of any shade, but I don't really think it's a solution for men whose dark-brown hair is going gray. Sometimes the contrast between dark hair and overlightened strands really makes a man look older rather than younger. I'll tell you more about my feelings on dark hair that's graying later on—and I do have strong personal feelings on this subject.

There are other problems with streaking or frosting. To achieve the streaks you must use a bleaching agent, which changes the texture of the hair that's streaked. So now you are dealing with two different types of hair, which causes conditioning and even styling snags. In addition, when highlighting isn't done properly, the effect is garish, overstated, rather like an elegant car gone wrong by too many flamboyant accessories, rally stripes and the like.

There are two methods for highlighting. Usually the at-home kits include a cap with holes through which the strands of hair are pulled for lightening. The second technique involves picking out specific strands to be bleached and then wrapping them in aluminum foil to separate them from the rest of the hair. The foil provides a surer approach to the lightening than a cap, which makes it hard to determine just which strands and how much hair to lighten.

The process is very tricky, and although you may be able to pull it off attractively on your own at home (or with some loving help) the first or second time, after that you run into all kinds of difficulties with overbleaching, oxidation and the rest, so don't make it a habit. If your hair is a medium shade of brown or lighter, borrow a tip from even the youngest teenage girl with similarly colored hair: apply the juice of one lemon to your hair and sit in the sun for half an hour; the effect will be very natural streaking.

Semipermanent Hair Color

Hair-coloring products labeled "semipermanent" are very gentle and "soft penetrating," and don't require the aid of a peroxide developer. The hair color produced by such products fades gradually and naturally, usually after five shampoos or so. Semipermanent color is recommended for those who want to try out a shade for the first time and are wary about a permanent tint—either because they are not sure of what they want or because they are apprehensive of the results. These products are good for covering gray hair (and removing the yellow stains, caused by pollution, nicotine and other residues), and for younger men who want to deepen or add highlights to their natural color.

Semipermanent coloring is rather easy and safe to do on your own. The results are very natural-looking and the color never rubs off on linens or clothing. Touch-ups aren't necessary because a new application is repeated every four weeks. In addition, the condition of the hair is generally improved after each application by the grace of beneficial "fillers" added to the formulas.

Temporary Rinses or Tints

There isn't a man over thirty around who hasn't heard of Grecian Formula and hasn't seen the TV scenario. The executive is up for a big meeting, but upon looking in his mirror one morning, realizes he doesn't look as young or as dynamic as some of the other company go-getters. The solution: fade down that gray with a few deft applications of Grecian Formula, and in doing so reestablish his image as an energetic, very-much-in-his-prime mover and shaker.

Well, in the first place, we all know that it takes a little more than hair color to change an image. More important, however, is that if you decide a color change is in order, you're probably better off with permanent or semipermanent coloring, which doesn't have to be reapplied every few days—the case with temporary rinses, tints or "coaters," such as Grecian Formula. If you're opting for a change, choose the simplest, most enduring, least bothersome approach, one that won't wash out every time you wash your hair.

Which Color Is Right for You?

Now you know the methods you can use to change the color of your hair, but the most important point is determining the color that's correct for you. You can't just make a blanket statement and say, "I want my hair to look the way it did when I was twenty-five." When you were twenty-five and a heartbreaking Al Pacino type, your dark hair looked right with your complexion. A quarter of a century later, however, that same near-black hair will be much too harsh for your skin and face and will, in fact, make you look older.

A good rule of thumb is, the darker your hair color, the younger you should be. The older you are, the lighter your hair coloring should be. Even nature is helpful in making our hair lighter as we mature. And personally, I never fight Mother Nature. Certainly with all the best products at my fingertips, and top professional colorists to make any transformation I desire, it would be very simple for me to turn my graying hair back to its original brown.

But I would never do this, even though I like to look as young as the next man. My skin pigmentation is very different now than it was when I was twenty, and unless really carefully orchestrated, as I've said many times in this chapter, most artificial color looks just like what it is—artificial. There are some well-known men out there in the world who feel the same way. Think of Cary Grant and how marvelous he looks; gray hair only adds to his image as a romantic charmer. Look at Prince Rainier of Monaco, whose silver hair has made him look, not older, but more dignified and commanding. Paul Newman, more than half a century old now, is not about to color his hair, and the streaks of silver actually serve to highlight his legendary blue eyes.

"Well," you say, "I'm convinced. I won't try to hide the gray. But my hair doesn't look like Cary Grant's or Prince Rainier's. It just looks old and dull." There are rinses on the market which are supposed to polish the silver, but I've found that in time these products create a streaky, tarnished look. In addition, if you smoke, or if you're around smokers, a rinse seems to grab more nicotine from the air and ends up giving hair a yellowish tint. Keep your hair in top condition, clean and nourished, and the gray will sparkle on its own.

By now I may have offended many readers who are feeling that, Cary Grant and Prince Rainier and George Michael notwithstanding, a new color is called for. By all means go ahead, and you can get your new color one of two ways: at a salon or at home. Keep these points in mind.

Why Choose a Salon?

After twenty-five years of experience, I have to tell you that it's almost impossible to do correct hair coloring at home. And I base that not only on what I know is right but also on all the home-colored jobs that I've seen go wrong. For one thing, you can't take your hair, put it on a block and stand over it while you color it.

Not only can a professional colorist stand behind you and above you and eliminate all the physical difficulties of the chore encountered when you do it yourself, but more important, he understands colors, chemicals and how to put them all together for the best results. A new hair color should be designed with foresight: a colorist should be able to determine how the hair will look ten or twenty years from now if he has to gradually keep lightening it. A good colorist knows, for example, that hair color should *not* be matched to facial tones, but should be keyed to the color of the inside forearm from the wrist to the elbow. Although the face can be altered by aging or suntan, forearm tones always remain the same and are the best barometer for compatible color.

As for maintaining the color once you've changed it, again professionals are the best solution for quality results. If, however, for financial or time reasons you can't continue professional coloring, then at least you can benefit from the *initial* professional treatment. The color choice and the way the treatment is done can act as a future guide to help you maintain your hair better when and if you color it yourself.

More Rules to Remember for At-Home Coloring

1. *Always do a patch test.* This is extremely important, especially when you're using a product for the first time. Use a cotton ball to remove any natural oils from behind your ear or in the crook of your elbow and then apply a dab of the coloring product. If, within twenty-four hours, you experience any breaking out or itching, take an antihistamine (Allerest is fine), drink plenty of liquids, wash the experimental area off well—and throw out the stuff! Don't skip this important patch test: allergic reactions can be devastating.

2. *Work with dirty hair.* Always use hair color or bleach on hair in its soiled state. It's a mistake to shampoo it first, contrary to directions on most do-it-yourself products. The oil that builds up between shampoos actually protects the skin against the unwanted invasion of chemicals into the system. It's one thing to color your *hair,* quite another to put those chemicals into your body via the unprotected skin. In fact, the morning before coloring your hair, don't even brush it!

3. *Don't fight the red in your hair.* Amateur colorists make the mistake

of trying to eliminate any red pigmentation. But red pigment is an important factor in the actual structure of the hair. If you try to remove this color via overtinting or bleaching, you remove the last link that holds the chain reaction of the hair itself together. And more, red highlights are good and flattering, so exploit them, don't eliminate them.

4. *Learn how often to color.* The primary rule is, avoid overlapping of color by retouching surfaces only every *four weeks*. No more and no less. Exactly every four weeks. If dyeing or bleaching is scheduled sooner, you overprocess the previously treated hair and this is very noticeable from the hair's dry and brittle appearance. If you color or bleach five or six weeks later, you *underlap* the previously treated hair and create an uneven structure of the hair. This is harmful since the original chemical process of dyeing or bleaching altered the structure of the hair to begin with. So an exact four-week retouch is a must.

In addition, after coloring, you must allow your hair to remain dry for three days and three nights to allow the process to oxidize properly.

Colored Hair Calls for Special Care

Remember that bleached or dyed hair does not possess the resilient qualities of virgin hair, and therefore you have to be more careful about exposing it to harmful elements and chemicals. For example, if your hair has been bleached or highlighted and then you swim in a chlorine-treated swimming pool every day for three months as part of your fitness routine, you could end up being a close facsimile of the boy with green hair, because the chemical reaction to the copper in the water, when combined with the bleaching chemicals, can add up to this disaster. If you've covered up the gray in your dark-brown hair, swimming in this same pool may result in your hair's turning a shade somewhere between dirty pewter and a twenty-year-old copper penny, again because of the chemicals in the pool in combination with the chemicals in your hair.

One more thing: dyed or bleached or highlighted hair requires about double the amount of conditioners and special treatments as untouched, untreated hair and naturally cannot take as much abuse. In this vein, if your overall look depends on using a blowdryer or other electrical appliance, you'd better make sure you use such a gadget for the shortest time possible and as infrequently as possible.

The Why, What and How of Permanents

Let's say you have board-straight, fine hair that always looks as if it should be styled in the same Buster Brown hairdo our mother used to be so good (or so bad) at achieving twenty years ago. You might be a perfect candidate for a body wave (really a permanent wave) and today you would be among many, many men to have one—and not at all the exception.

The permanent wave, although originally and specifically designed for women, can conquer many of the problems men have with hair that just won't stay put.

Before I tell you why you should have one and what the beneficial effects might be, I think you should know what a permanent really is, and how it works.

A Man Started It All

Seventy-five years ago a German hairdresser named Charles Nessler was trying to figure out how and why naturally curly hair was naturally curly. He discovered that straight hair is round like a pencil or a strand of spaghetti and wavy hair is flat, like a ribbon, which accounts for its ability to curl or wave. He also realized that if you wet hair with water and wind it around a finger or a roller (what we know as a setting), this stretches the outside of the hair and changes its molecular structure so that it more closely resembles curly hair.

But in order to change the hair *permanently,* it was necessary to penetrate the hair with some chemical solution, curl it as if for setting and then stamp that set into the hair once and for all with the use of an agent that would establish a built-in memory, so the hair would "remember" that curl. Nessler experimented for years and in 1905, in London, he perfected what became the first permanent, causing a sensation among those women who are always willing to try the latest thing to be and remain more beautiful.

His technique was introduced to Americans as early as 1908. First he softened the hair with a borax solution. Now think about that: this is the same chemical we know as 20 Mule Team borax, so praised for its superjanitorial properties. Then, when the hair was soaked with this "wonder worker," it was wound around a rod (actually, a small roller), from the scalp to the ends.

The third step was the application of heat. The inventive Nessler, at this point, had to rely on irons heated over a gas burner. He would carefully heat the curled strand for a short amount of time, then go on to the next strand of hair. Soak it with borax, wind on a rod, heat for a few minutes, and so on. Initially, then, to have a permanent, only one curl at a time could be done, which made for hours of misery in the vein of "You must suffer to be beautiful."

Eventually Nessler invented an electric heater that could cover the entire head at once—not that this cut down on the suffering; it simply made the painful duration shorter. Now after the borax soaking, every strand of hair was wound on rods, and then these rods were connected to a dreadful-looking machine that would cook the whole mess for an hour or so.

There were drawbacks, of course. Aside from the possibility of electric shock when the permanent was administered by less than skilled technicians; aside from the heavy weight of all those rods and wires; and aside from the probability of a good deal of hair loss due to breakage from the strong chemicals used, the results were not tremendously appealing. The hair was curly, yes—but sometimes so curly (in fact, kinky), that the poor victim would hide her hair behind hats or scarves or turbans for a month or two until the perm settled down and became workable.

By the 1930s, this situation changed. Early in that decade improvements were made in the solutions and in the hardware which made the heat permanent a less dubious adventure. But the major breakthrough occurred in 1934 when A. F. Willat, an engineer who probably hated the way his wife's hair looked, developed the *cold-wave permanent,* a process used almost universally throughout the world today. In fact, we still use Willat end papers on modern permanents. Hardware was completely eliminated: while having a permanent you no longer had to look like a refugee from a space-age torture chamber on *Buck Rogers* or *Star Trek.*

The cold-wave permanent depends solely on chemicals, and not only are the results much more predictable, but the process is much more comfortable to go through.

The key word, of course is *chemicals.* And although it's possible today to get magnificent results with permanenting, remember that any chemical application changes the natural structure of the hair. Remember, too, that in the case of permanenting, women were the guinea pigs; they went through all the experimentation (quite adventurously and courageously, as a matter of fact), all the kinks (if you will allow me a pun), until the procedure was ironed out. Today, if you opt for a permanent, although you are taking the risk of having chemicals applied to your hair, you're not taking the same kind of risks—in terms of either chemicals or degrees of chance—that women have been taking since Nessler started fooling around more than seventy-five years ago.

So, taking your own courage in hand, this is what happens when you have a permanent:

How Is a Permanent Done?

The four steps involved in chemical hair waving are presoftening and winding; softening; hardening; unwinding, combing and brushing out.

I Presoftening and Winding

The first major point is that before winding on circular rods (simply another version of rollers), the hair has to be presoftened. In my salon we always presoften with plain water, *not* a waving solution. It stands to reason that if you presoften with a waving preparation, the side of the hair which was wound first will eventually turn out to be wavier than the side which was wound last.

And imagine the terrible results if the operator who is winding your hair gets a phone call from her babysitter, or absolutely must take a bathroom break in the middle of the winding. The length of time the operator is away can make a very drastic difference in the finished product. Then, too, the length of your hair dictates how long and how many rollers will be necessary, and this can throw off the predicted expectations if you're using a chemical solution instead of plain water.

On the positive side, the water used to wind the rollers will act as an activator for the waving solution and you will have a better permanent in the long run.

II Softening

After the winding of the hair has been completed, the hair must be softened with a special solution to break the structural cross bonds of the hair. This is left on the rolled-up hair for five or ten minutes, depending on the structure, thickness and curling goal in mind, so that after the bonds break they will assume their new position in terms of the designed waving pattern. This is known as the *processing time*. It's up to the operator, who has studied the condition of your hair and done a preliminary "test curl," and who knows the strength of the waving solution to determine how long this processing time should be.

III   Hardening

Before the rods are removed and your hair is released from that "waving pattern" formed by the rods, it's essential to mend those broken cross bonds, to fix them in their new position for all time—that is, until enough hair grows out so that you are a candidate for another perm. If your hair is removed from the rods before this hardening takes place, the permanent waving will be a complete failure. Hardening is achieved by a combination of drying the hair and the application of still more chemicals called *neutralizers*.

It's important to note here that if the softening of the hair has been overdone (i.e., if the waving solution has been left on too long), the hardening stage won't produce the wave either. The reason for this is that overexposure of the hair to chemicals has damaged it, causing the chains of keratin to break. If this occurs, then the hair must go through a veritable R & R period, a rest-and-recuperation time, in order to restore the hair health completely before exposing it once again to chemicals.

IV   Unwinding, Brushing and Combing Out

After the new bonds are established, your hair is released by unwinding the rods. The curls that were formed will be a little bit tighter than the desired finished result. But this is a planned curliness to facilitate the creation of a definite style.

For the finished product, your hair is then set in a preplanned way, using regular setting rollers instead of the smaller permanent-wave rods. Then the set is dried as usual, ending with the brushing out and combing of the desired hairstyle. The end product should be soft and natural-looking and should make the maintenance of your hairstyle much easier than before. That doesn't mean that you have to set your hair from now on, but the first time after a permanent, setting the hair is a must.

Some Permanent Considerations

Now you know how it's done. But is a permanent the right move for you? Consider these factors:

How Long Is Your Hair?

Permanents are best applied to hair that is six to nine or twelve inches long. (One reason I often discourage permanents for women with very long hair, and, of course, these are my favorite customers, is that it tends to kink up, which defeats the purpose of the permanent wave itself when what you want is a curl, or body, not a kink.) Ironically, then, men are among the *best* candidates for a body permanent because their hair is usually no more than six inches in length.

Since hair grows half an inch a month, within a year your hair will have grown six inches. Any damaging results of a permanent will by then have grown out and you can repeat the process all over again, starting fresh, as it were. (A woman with twelve-inch, "two-year-old" hair would have a lot more problems than you with your new, "virgin" hair.)

How Much Body Do You Want?

The size of the rod used determines the size of the final wave or curl. Small rods spaced one-half to one inch apart will produce very curly results; for a body wave, which is actually the same thing as a permanent, the rods are larger and are placed one inch to two inches apart. At this point, I should explain what a body wave really means. If you curl three hairs, they will occupy twice as much space; in other words, they will have more *body* than three straight hairs. It is this kind of "positioning" of the hair into a wavy stage that makes it appear thicker.

A current fad in men's hairstyling is to have a permanent which gives the effect of an afro, euphemistically called a "natural look." While I don't recommend this for every man, in some cases, where a man has naturally curly and fine hair which is difficult to maintain in a smoothed-down style, by having a body wave the hair looks more luxuriant, looks "natural," and is much easier to care for. But hair that has been permanented in this style has only about one-half to one-third the strength of normal hair; it is difficult to comb and more likely to break in the combing process, and it's drier than usual; it has to be treated very carefully, tenderly. (Avoid blowdrying; whenever possible let your hair dry naturally.)

What Time of the Year Is It?

The degree of curl will also be dictated by the season of the year. For example, if you're a very outdoorsy type, don't permanent your hair just before summer unless you want an afro look. If you're a bookworm, however, who never sets foot on an Atlantic (or Pacific) beach, it's better to permanent your hair at the start of summer because this will give you more body.

In addition, the ultraviolet rays of the sun will produce changes in the cortex of the hair. If you like the outdoor life, your permanent will have a shorter life span. The best temperature for the most optimum life expectancy of a permanent is cool to mild weather with average humidity. If you're going to spend a great deal of time outdoors, wear a hat and pay extra attention to conditioners to keep your hair in the best state. (And, of course, because hair grows half an inch per month, every time you have a haircut you'll be cutting off some of the permanented hair, thus reducing the permanent's life span.)

Other Influences on Your Permanent

Diet

Natural hair growth, as you know by now, is greatly influenced by the food you eat, especially in relation to sulfur-containing amino acids. Some diets lack the necessary top-grade proteins, and if the amount of sulfur provided is not sufficient to promote healthy hair growth, your hair might not be able to support the permanent as long as it should.

Medicines

Not infrequently, sulfur is used in the formulation of internal medicines and drugs. This sulfur, which then circulates in your blood, may be responsible for arrested hair growth as well as continued nervous tension and stress. All or one of these factors can change the chemical structure of your hair and account for how it responds to the application of permanent-wave chemicals.

Hormonal Imbalances

Natural aging, the aftereffects of certain illnesses and so on can produce hormonal disturbances which in turn can promote changes in the hair's cortex. These ultimately can cause failures of permanent waves or a shorter life span of a perm due to conditions already present in the hair shaft before the operator even began to soften your hair in preparation for a permanent.

The Do-It-Yourself Varieties

There are miracles of hair-waving products on the market today, meant for either professional or amateur use. At this point I have to remind you of the meaning of *amateur*. That is, literally, a person who engages in a pursuit for pleasure (because he or she *loves* to, from the Latin *amare,* to love), or a person who is not an expert.

If you love yourself and you like your hair, your best bet is to leave chemical processes to the *experts,* who know what they are dealing with. After reading this book, you may be an expert amateur at understanding your hair—and you should be, or I've failed in my goal —but you will also know that some hair care tasks are better left to the professionals.

I have a boat, my very favorite material possession, I suppose, and I like to think I am a loving and knowledgeable amateur in terms of the boat, the *Nubi II.* I am proud of my ability to maneuver the *Nubi* in and out of her slip; I am confident when it comes to refurbishing my *Nubi;* I even understand the engine and the carburetor and the ram's horns and the transducers. But I understand them *just enough* to know when I have real trouble that it's time for the experts to take over from the amateur.

There is nothing wrong in admitting that professionals can do a better job than you can.

Now that I've hit you pretty heavily on this, I will give you a few cautions should you decide to try your own hand at a home permanent, or even enlist the support of a willing assistant.

1. Please read the directions not once, not twice but at least three times before you dive in. Always do a test curl to determine how your hair will react to the chemicals, just as a professional would in a salon. Try to do not only the test curl but the entire permanent in a *moderate* temperature of from 68 to 72 degrees F., which is the temperature the perm was originally developed for. Any hotter than that will make the

permanent take faster; a colder environment will mean the waving needs a longer "take."

2. Never try to achieve two chemical transformations at once. If you are going to color your hair or bleach it, schedule a permanent at least two weeks before. The permanent should always be done *first*. And then choose a coloring or bleaching product meant for permanented hair.

3. If you've botched up the job, don't compensate by trying again. Please wait until the damaged hair grows out—or cut it off. The overuse of such harsh chemicals can only spell disaster.

The Straight and Harrowing Path

In all the years that I've worked so closely with women, I've always been impressed by their daring, their adventurous spirit in the realm of self-improvement. If I were to give out medals for bravery, the top awards would go to women who straighten their hair—for that is certainly a perilous course to take.

Many men and women think that hair straightening involves the same process as a permanent. This is not entirely true. A permanent *stretches* the bonds of the hair via use of chemicals and winding the hair on rods. There is no exertion of *pull*. In straightening, after chemicals are applied, the hair is combed through to straighten it—a procedure that involves pull which can't really be measured and is much less controllable than permanenting. And believe me, I have seen some nightmarish results of straightening (especially when done at home) in which it might almost have been better if somone had removed all the hair and started fresh, from scratch.

Clearly, I'm not in favor of straightening (either done *chez vous* or professionally). It is almost impossible to try to uncurl curly hair permanently without serious damage. Straightening, you must realize, is akin to bleaching in the sense that it must be repeated at regular intervals. Within a year or two, continued straightening will take its toll—a price far too expensive to pay for the short-range advantages.

There are other problems with straightening, in case you need more reasons to be convinced. Coarse hair is easier to straighten because it's strong (but coarse hair is never as curly, anyway); fine hair, the type which tends to be the kinkiest, is also much more delicate and can never be truly straight anyway. In the latter instance, all you can do is remove some of the kink. At the same time, straightening also removes any kind of "holding power," so that you may be left with very fine limp, stubborn, "nothing" hair that you can't do a thing with anyway.

The question of virgin hair is also a factor in how safe it is to straighten. If you've had bleaching or coloring, then you really multiply the dangers of using chemical straighteners. You may have to decide on one alternative to another: do you want your hair to have a more vibrant color? Or do you want some built-in body via a permanent? Don't try to have your cake and eat it, too.

Taming Wiry, Curly Hair

It's difficult to keep the curl out of short hair, especially during humid weather. I've noticed more men wearing natural frizzies during the summertime, and although I personally don't like the look, I know this makes warm-weather hair care a great deal easier.

During any season, however, curly hair can be made more manageable and more easily controlled if it is cut all one length, not in steps. Even a crew cut will be less curly if it's cut three inches *all over*. Another way of straightening short curly hair was taught to me by one of my few short-haired female clients who was in the process of growing her hair long. Angela always brushes her hair *against* the grain, and although she's now on the way to a totally different way of dealing with her hair, when it was four or five inches long, this method helped her tame her hair. After a vigorous brushing in the opposite direction of how she wanted to wear it, she found she could slick it down in uncurly styles.

Chapter Seven

What's in a Hair?

By now you've learned a great deal about how to care for your hair and how to stimulate circulation through massage and exercise. The emphasis has been on what to do so that your hair *looks* better. Men (and women) don't like to think about the health aspects of hair unless they have a severe problem—excessive fallout, or dandruff, or dryness. For the most part, people abuse their hair, and then expect miracles overnight when they finally do consult a specialist.

Doctors or trichologists (a formal name for hair specialists) can help, of course. But you can sidestep many of the problems by understanding the "nature of the beast," by knowing that most of the characteristics of your hair were predestined long before you were a twinkle, or whatever, in your parents' eyes. Then, armed with this knowledge, you have to understand what you can or can't expect from your hair.

As a scientist, I've always been fascinated by the structure of hair. It's so thin, for example (the average male hair is 1/525 to 1/300 of an inch; the average female hair is 1/500 to 1/250 of an inch), yet so strong: it has been scientifically proven that hair is stronger than a copper wire of the same diameter, and that one hair will hold a weight of approximately five to seven ounces. Under a microscope hair is fascinating, but maybe you want to say, "So what? I'm not a scientist. I don't care about the sex life of earthworms, so why should I care how my hair looks magnified five hundred times?" But you *should* care because a look at a magnified section of hair will tell you why you have a lot of problems—or, happily, why you don't.

You know that saying, you can't grow hair on a golf ball? It's true. Hair will grow only when follicles—small pockets in the skin—are present. These hair-sources-to-be begin forming when a fetus is only a few weeks old. Three months before birth, every hair follicle you'll ever have has already been formed. Almost the entire surface of the skin is covered with hair follicles, but most remain dormant and never produce hair. (The only truly naked parts of the body are the palms of the hands, the soles of the feet, the lips and the nipples.)

The follicles on your scalp are extremely active, though, and produce abundant hair: one of a baby's first gifts to his parents is often a lush head of wiry hair (which he loses a few weeks later so he can join the universal ranks of infant Winston Churchill look-alikes). Other follicles develop only at certain times in life, such as those of the hair that arrives under the arms and in the pubic area with the onset of puberty.

Hair follicles are bunched on the scalp in uneven groups of two to five follicles each; sometimes two follicles grow together and it seems as if two or three hairs are growing out of one follicle. While you rush through your own life cycle, each follicle is following a life cycle of its own, producing hair for about two to four years, then taking a short vacation before busily resuming hair production. During the active period the new growth pushes out the older part of the hair farther and farther away from the *papilla* until it falls out.

The papilla is a very vital part of each follicle, a small "outgrowth" of skin shaped like a doorknob and lying at the bottom of each follicle. The neck of the doorknob is the narrowest part. The papilla not only contains blood vessels to supply nourishment to the hair but it dictates a lot of characteristics about that hair.

The pattern of cell growth at the papilla, for example, will determine whether you have straight, wavy or curly hair. Straight hair, of course, is the most common, but when the growth pattern of the papilla is uneven the result will be curly hair, which usually reaches its peak during adolescence and tends to tame down as we grow older. Moreover, the cell pattern can change with circumstances (illness, drugs, diet, pregnancy) that can cause the hair to become board straight at certain times. Kinky hair is another pattern caused by changes in the nature of the papilla.

So the follicle and its very important component, the papilla, start the hair on its way. The hair grows—before birth and for exactly fifteen minutes after death, as a matter of fact. (Although hair and nails are made of the same material, nails grow on a cadaver for six to eight months, sometimes two years, but nobody knows why.)

Hair is made of strong elastic strands of fibrous protein called *keratin* and is composed of oxygen, iron, nitrogen, hydrogen, sulfur, carbon and phosphorus. The exact proportions of these elements vary with the sex, age, hair type and color of hair. What makes hair so strong and resistant to outside influences is probably the relatively high sulfur content—from 4 to 8 percent. (Skin contains much less sulfur; that's why it wrinkles and is more susceptible to harsh chemicals. Naturally red hair has the highest amount of sulfur and is the strongest hair type.)

If you pull a hair out of your scalp and then look at it, you'll see a small bit of white tissue, which is actually part of the follicle that has broken away. But that's about all you'll see. A hair looks like a hair, a single strand of fiber. But under a microscope you would observe that hair is constructed in three different layers: the *shingle,* or *cuticle,* the *cortex* and the *medulla.*

The Cuticle, or Shingle

When magnified, the outside of your hair looks very much like the scales on a fish: the outer layer of the hair shaft is made up of hard, flattened, horny scales that overlap each other so that usually five or six or seven scales are arranged in order, giving the hair a strong and flexible network. Just as scales protect a fish, this layer protects the hair and also allows chemical changes (such as the absorption of color or of permanent waving) to take place. A key part of the scales is the orderly arrangement, or imbrications, of the tips, which point upward and outward in the direction of hair growth. If you rub a hair between your fingers lengthwise, your fingers will slide smoothly all the way to the ends, but if you slide your fingers in the opposite direction (against the "grain" of the imbrications), they won't move as smoothly. You are fighting the pattern of the shingles.

The cuticle acts as a guard dog, a protector of the second layer of the hair shaft—the cortex—from injury. If the cuticle is damaged through chemicals or improper care, then the cortex is exposed to danger or damage. When the cuticle breaks or dislodges at the end of the hair, the result is known as "split ends," a particularly irritating problem for women who are trying to let their hair grow long.

The cuticle also plays a part in determining whether your hair is dry, normal or oily. Tiny pockets in the scales hold the necessary supply of sebum, the natural oil of the scalp produced by the sebaceous glands. Sebum actually protects your hair from extremes of temperature and humidity, drying shampoos, chemical treatments and foreign elements that can be damaging. When there isn't enough sebum the hair and scalp will be dry and show a flaking condition similar to dandruff (but, unlike some cases of dandruff, this isn't contagious). Too much oil production causes oily hair and scalp conditions requiring frequent shampoos and the frustration of dealing with hard-to-manage, stringy, limp hair. The right amount of sebum gives your hair that nice gloss and sheen and enables you to claim "normal" hair.

The Cortex

This second layer is the most essential and accounts for between 75 and 90 percent of the bulk of your hair. The cortex controls how your hair behaves and determines properties of strength, elasticity, pliability, direction and growth patterns, width, quality and texture. The cortex is formed by millions of hard keratin fibers placed in a parallel position. Sometimes the fibers are twisted around each other, with the appearance (under a microscope) of heavy rope.

The cortex also holds the key to what color hair you'll have and *how much* you'll have. This layer is home for four natural pigments: black, brown, yellow and red; the variations in natural shades come about not only by the combinations of pigments but also by the type of pigment, the difference in pigment granules and air spaces in the cortex. With the exception of pure black oriental hair, most color gradations are based on different pigment combinations. Brown hair, the most common hair color, ranges in shades from blondish brown and reddish brown to darkest brown, when combined with black pigment.

Blond hair, of course, is predominantly yellow, but even then it has some red or brown pigment. Blond hair is the most changeable shade and is based on the weakest pigment. As one ages, the other colors tend to take over and the formerly blond child becomes an average light-brown-haired adult. Even red hair is mixed with black to result in rust or copper shades, or brown or yellow tints, which produce lighter, "strawberry-blond" hair.

There is a relationship, too, between hair color and hair quantity: blonds are most blessed with an average of 140,000 hairs; redheads average about 110,000; men or women with brown hair have 75,000 hairs and people with black hair have the least, a paltry 60,000 hairs.

The Medulla

This inner core of soft keratin is formed by a column of cells either two or four rows in width, but not everyone has this layer; it can be broken or entirely absent (often because of certain drugs or medications). However, hair that lacks a medulla is no worse than hair *with* a medulla—one of science's mysteries; one of the body's vestigial remains.

How Much Is Enough?

Here you are now with your 60,000 or 75,000 or 110,000 or 140,000 hairs (each with its cuticle, cortex and, possibly, medulla) and suddenly you begin to notice some of these precious possessions are on your comb or in the sink or on your shoulder or on the pillowcase instead of on your head. And you panic.

Don't worry.

It's normal to shed from 50 to 80 hairs a day, and it's normal for each of those hairs to be replaced by the hardworking follicles, some resting, some active. On any given day 90 percent of the hair is in the growing (*anagen*) stage, which lasts about a thousand days and 10 percent is in the resting (*telogen*) period, which lasts about a hundred days. In the resting stage the follicle weakens and eventually the shaft comes out, resulting in that normal loss of 50 to 80 hairs daily. Interestingly, most of this fallout occurs in the morning.

The length of your hair is a factor, too. Although 50 to 80 hairs a day is the normal range of loss, a head that's cut in a crew cut may lose 87 hairs a day; hair twelve inches in length could suffer the loss of maybe 26 hairs a day. If your hair is healthy the 50 or 80 or 26 hairs lost will be replaced by an equal amount of new hairs.

In addition to day-to-day loss, we also shed more hair during six periods of our lives: from birth to the age of three, at ten, at twenty-two, around age twenty-six, at thirty-six and at fifty-four—all in relation to hormonal changes in our bodies and all very, very normal, and all in relation to the six inches of hair (one-half inch per month) which we all grow every year.

Hair also changes as we age, and in fact, by the time we are octogenarians we will have thinner hair to show for our years: some of those follicles just stop functioning. Actually, the maximum hair growth for men occurs between the ages of twenty-two and thirty-six (women enjoy the most luxuriant hair growth between the ages of fifteen and thirty), and there is some evidence that hair (and nails) grow faster in summer than in winter, but this difference is so slight it can hardly be measured.

How to Measure Fallout

If you're worried about hair loss for any of the reasons cited in this chapter, here's how to tell whether your hair loss is normal or whether you should see a hair specialist. Take ten envelopes and date them consecutively from the first of January to the tenth, for example. Each day put the hair that falls out into the corresponding envelope. Then, two months later, date another ten envelopes from the first to the tenth of the month and repeat the procedure. At the end of the sixty-day period you'll be able to see whether your hair fallout has increased or decreased. Remember, though, that fifty to eighty lost hairs a day is absolutely normal.

There's another test, too: if the roots look like round doorknobs, usually the loss is from normal molting. If four or five hairs have a bulbous root that looks like a miniature scallion, you had better see a doctor or a trichologist because you may be experiencing permanent fallout.

The point is, some daily hair loss is normal. If the amount in your sink basin suddenly seems excessive for several days or weeks (take time out and count the fallen hairs), you may have something to worry about—which I'll explain in the next chapter.

Chapter Eight

The Bald Truth

Although I have been stressing the point that some hair fallout every day is perfectly normal, many men and women panic if they see twenty or so hairs in their comb or sink. And there's nothing new or modern about this; the alarm has sounded ever since man discovered there was more to living than surviving.

Because hair loss is so traumatic, men and women alike all through history have been ready victims to the charlatans who have promised hair growth. A four-thousand-year-old Egyptian papyrus cited a hair potion for women made from such exotic substances as toe of dog, refuse of date and hoof of ass. For men the prescription called for equal parts of lion, hippopotamus, crocodile, ibex, goose and snake. In ancient Rome there were dozens of lotions and potions, to apply or to drink, but none of these grew one extra hair on the head of Julius Caesar. Fortunately for him, the laurel wreath which he wore as a sign of grandeur and leadership also camouflaged his baldness.

In more modern times, the snake-oil entrepreneurs sold many

types of miracle hair restorers which were worthless unless you drank them to enjoy the alcoholic content—and many people did. All the hair salves, balms, elixirs and other preparations perfected and promoted through the centuries have one thing in common: they can't grow hair for a person suffering from serious thinning or balding.

Excessive fallout (either temporary or permanent) is called *alopecia,* but before I get into the different types of alopecia I must remind you that genes count—as they do in determining anything from one's I.Q. to one's possible longevity. We literally inherit our hair from our mother's father and our father's mother, along with any of their hair problems; hair will be thicker, thinner, sparse or abundant, straight or curly, depending on your family tree. We can also inherit directly from parents such diseases as diabetes and thyroid deficiencies or excesses, two real threats to hair health.

Temporary Alopecia, or Baldness, Can Result from:

Trauma

Trauma results from outward stress. Traction alopecia, for example can be the "reward" for women who pull their hair into ponytails or chignons year after year. But trauma can also stem from excessive heat, friction, strong hair preparations (dyes and bleaches), X rays and major surgery, all of which extract a toll from the hair.

Traumatic spot baldness can also come about by a severe blow to the head. About ten years ago, for example, a mechanic with very thick, dark brown hair was working on my boat when I unexpectedly jumped aboard and scared him and he accidently banged the back of his head against the engine starter. Six weeks later he had a bald spot about the size of a fifty-cent piece. Knowing my background in hair care, he came to me and asked why. I remembered his accident and sent him to a dermatologist for cortisone injections. In four months and four days, the hair had grown back and he still enjoys a full, luxuriant head of hair.

Cortisone is not always necessary with traumatic baldness, however. The teenage daughter of my co-author was celebrating her own team's victory at softball when she was hit on the head by a foul-tipped hardball while watching her brother's Little League game. She fell and struck her head on one of the spectators' benches. She suffered a concussion, which, fortunately, wasn't serious, but a few weeks later she noticed that she had a dime-sized bald spot on the top of her scalp where she had hit the grandstand. Maria is young and healthy and her hair is young and healthy, too, and without the benefit of cortisone, her hair grew back within four months and four days. Specifically, *four months and four days,* an astonishing but always accurate timetable!

In each of these cases, correcting the condition, and cortisone therapy (when it's medically indicated) can usually reverse the hair loss. Not infrequently, however, the resultant hair growth is completely different in texture. There have been many instances where people with curly hair—in fact, kinky hair—have found that after injections of cortisone the hair grew in stronger and almost straight in texture. (Cortisone, of course, is prescribed only in case of serious medical problems, so one can't look to this hormone as a way of straightening out curly hair.)

Local Infections

Bacterial, viral or fungus dermatological infections can cause spot fallout and may have to be treated with ultraviolet rays, cortisone ointments or medicated shampoos.

General Infections

Infections involving high fevers, flu, scarlet fever, pneumonia, can result in hair loss about two months after the illness; other diseases, including syphilis and cancer take their toll on hair health. In many European countries, the hair is still automatically and drastically cut off on patients with such diseases. This, of course, does not affect the health of the hair, nor does it encourage regrowth, but it does remove any germs that may be lodged in the hair. Cutting hair during illness is an old-fashioned idea, with no basis in medical fact.

Chemicals or Drugs

Antibiotics, chemotherapy and cortisone (and this is ironic, since cortisone injections can often arrest and correct spot fallout) can result in hair loss, usually temporary, unless the condition is grave, as with cancer, and drug therapy must be continued despite the side effects.

Environmental or Emotional Stress

Field workers and peasants have better hair than urban dwellers and executives, not only because of less tension but also because they enjoy a healthier environment. You can make the generalization that people who work mainly with their hands instead of their brainpower will usually have better hair. In addition, personal problems—a broken heart, a checkbook constantly in the red, problems with children, the loss of a job—can all produce temporary hair loss, which usually abates once the emotional turmoil is settled.

When you're tense, the muscles in your scalp and neck tense up, too, restricting the flow of blood. Among my clients, I have almost a thousand physicians, Ph.D.s, psychologists, accountants, stockbrokers, advertising executives, actresses, models—all of whom are constantly under tension and pressure. In so many cases, when I examine their scalps, they are as tight as drums, squeezing the hair roots to pieces. To aid them, I developed the special scalp massage for eggheads I mentioned earlier in Chapter Two.

The Real Thing

We have been discussing temporary thinning or balding brought on by the special circumstances discussed above; permanent thinning or balding, however, is another story. Unless you can make being bald pay off handsomely in the grand manner of Yul Brynner and Telly Savalas, if you're a man you would rather have a full head of hair than not. As for women, there isn't one in the whole world (with the exception of Persis Khambatta, who starred in the first *Star Trek* movie) who would choose to be bald.

Yet millions of American men and, increasingly, women must spend a third or even a half of their lives with progressively thinning hair. There is a definite difference between baldness and increasing thinning. If a man or woman is bald, that's it. But thinning is a situation with greater ramifications.

If, for example, you are a dark-haired Latin or Mediterranean-type male who normally has about 60,000 hair roots, if you lose half those roots through fallout, this is a disaster. But if you are a fair-haired Swedish or Dutch-type blond with 140,000 roots and you lose 30,000, this is not a major loss: you still have 110,000 hairs left on your head. For this reason more dark-haired men are bald or balding than light-haired men.

But after a certain point, it's the hereditary change in hormones that affects all men who are going to be bald, whether they have blond, brown or red hair.

There is no mistaking the figures: 95 percent of permanent baldness in men and women is caused by hormonal, congenital and aging factors; the major hormonal culprit for both sexes is the male hormone, *androgen.*

We have told you that it is the female hormone, *estrogen,* that encourages hair growth. During puberty, and for several decades afterward, in most men the production of estrogen is balanced by the production of androgen (and another male hormone, progesterone). At about fifty-four, this hormonal balance shifts (yes, there is really such a condition as male menopause), men produce less estrogen and that is when most men begin to lose hair. In some cases thinning occurs much earlier, because of hereditary conditions and the very fact that since certain men have fewer hair roots to begin with any loss is much more noticeable.

In women, the normal ratio of hormones is one part androgen to eight parts estrogen. While hair loss affects only one out of seven women *before* menopause (a condition which my medical colleagues call *female androgenetic alopecia*), after menopause that figure changes to one out of two. Women are still producing the same amount of androgen (about two-thirds as much as men do) but much less estrogen. The result of this imbalance is often very serious hair loss. But in this book we are concerned with the hormonal problems of men, so for an in-depth discussion of what women can do to solve thinning and balding brought on by hormones, I refer you to my earlier book, *George Michael's Secrets for Beautiful Hair* (Doubleday, 1981).

The Where and How of Balding

Very few people bald evenly and neatly all over the head. Most balding occurs on top of the head. When the human being finally stood up on his hind legs, adjustments for walking on two legs were made, the spine straightened, the neck took a vertical instead of horizontal position, but no adjustments were made for the top of the head, which is robbed of vital blood circulation when the body is erect. Consequently, the normal area for losing hair is smack on top. Another reason we bald right on top is that the roots on top of the head grow straight up, from the left to the right side, but the roots all around the rest of the head face straight down. On top of the head there is often sebaceous "backfeed," where the sebaceous fluid, so helpful to hair strength, goes back into the root and often suffocates it. Therefore, the exchange of roots on the top of the head is seven times as fast as it is for hair on the back of the head.

In addition, men have a flat little muscle under the scalp which tightens up during the most virile years of human life, and this constant flexing (especially apparent in men who work with their brains alone instead of their hands) weakens the hair roots and·hastens their departure. (You may have noticed that after a man who has been bald for years retires, suddenly fuzz starts to sprout on that shiny bald scalp. This sometimes occurs because the tension in his life is dramatically reduced and that flat muscle is now relaxed, which allows some of those hair follicles which have been dormant for years to start producing again.)

Whether you're a man or a woman, the first thing you should do if you're experiencing excessive fallout is to consult an endocrinologist, who will run a battery of tests to see whether your hair loss is due to permanent or hereditary changes, or whether it can be helped by topical or internal therapy. You'll be given an SMA profile which includes thyroid, kidney, calcium, enzyme and liver tests.

Topical Hormone Injections

There's more to be done for women—good for them, unfortunate for men. For one thing, as my friend Dr. Robert Berger, assistant professor at Mount Sinai College of Medicine in New York, has noted, women don't usually show a bald spot on the top of their heads or a recession at the peaks of their foreheads; rather they show a thinning all over the scalp. Such women can be helped by estrogen replacement, if their doctors agree this is indicated, but a more simple, less risky technique is the application of injections of estrogen to the scalp, a process which can take two or three years depending on how much damage has been done before a doctor was consulted. This same amount of estrogen, injected into the scalp, could be feminizing to men, so this treatment isn't recommended or practical.

Dr. Norman Orentreich, who has pioneered so many break-throughs and is most famous for the development of the well-known hair transplant, believes that in the next decade an anti-androgen pill will be developed which men will be able to take to avert baldness without experiencing the serious side effects of taking estrogen.

Until that day men can take advantage of some other choices that range from transplants to toupees to replace the hair that's lost.

Chapter Nine

Cover Your Losses

The late and very talented actor Sir Cedric Hardwicke once said, "Baldness may indicate masculinity, but it diminishes one's opportunity to find out."

In this spirit, many men will seek to replace their hair for the sake of looking virile, through temporary or permanent means, sometimes at great cost and at great pain. Because baldness is a sore spot in terms of anyone's vanity, solutions for ending or alleviating baldness often have a ready audience. In this chapter, I'll tell you the positive approaches for dealing with hair loss, discuss the hair-replacement procedures that work and give you the simple (often painful and disappointing) facts about those techniques and remedies to avoid.

Hair Transplants

After three decades, transplants have proven to be the most effective method of hair replacement for men and women who can't be helped by hormone treatment. Dr. Norman Orentreich perfected this technique in the fifties and estimates that in the last twenty-five years he's performed more than 50,000 transplants. Although Dr. Orentreich has more than 4,000 transplant cases a year (10 percent of them women), all over the United States there are over three hundred dermatologists, plastic surgeons and other specialists who each perform about 250 transplants annually. Joey Bishop, Hugh Downs, hockey star Bobby Hull, Senator William Proxmire, Frank Sinatra and quite recently Jack Nicholson are among their clients.

Although hair transplanting is not a short and sweet procedure— you don't go in once and get it over with—it is not a serious surgical procedure either. But it is long and tedious and the patient must be patient. The scalp is divided into two areas: the donor area (usually the back of the head where the follicles are going strong) and the receptor area (the bald spot which will receive the transplant).

Here's how it works:

The patient gets a local anesthetic, and then a "punch" about $5/32$ of an inch in diameter is injected into the scalp at one of the donor points, stamping out an area about ¼ inch deep. This is called a "plug." Transplants aren't made with individual hairs but rather with small pieces of scalp, each carrying about six to ten hair follicles.

Next, using the same punch, a hairless section of the scalp is removed and discarded and the vacant space is filled with the hair-growing plug from the donor area. During each session about thirty to fifty such plugs are implanted; then a bandage is pressed over the scalp which remains on for two or three days. There's usually some swelling, which disappears within two days, and although the transplants can be itchy, no scratching is allowed.

After about ten days, the scabs fall off, followed by a loss of hair in the transplanted plugs. According to Dr. Orentreich, the follicles "rest" for ten to twenty weeks and then a "new generation of hair" starts to appear. After a transplant, a patient must lead a fairly calm life—no drinking, no strenuous exercise or shampooing or brushing for at least a week to ten days.

This is not the end of it, though. Most patients have transplants done in five or six sessions spread out over a period of six months to two or three years, all depending on the area to be covered, the life-style and tolerance of the individual and so on.

After a transplant the result will not necessarily be a thick, glorious full head of hair, but your appearance will be immeasurably improved. The important thing is to choose a doctor with a good reputation: look at photographs of his results, and even better, take the word-of-mouth endorsement of a friend who has been satisfied with his own transplanted hair. Although there have been some successful transplants of hair in identical twins, scientists have not been able to beat the rejection which takes place when plugs from strangers or even other relatives are transplanted. This makes it almost impossible for a bald person with a poor donor area to have a transplant—pubic hair and body hair aren't satisfactory—but doctors are working to beat the rejection problem, and such transplants may be possible in the next few years.

The Bilobe Flap

A very different technique of surgical hair replacement was developed almost two decades ago by a New York plastic surgeon, Dr. Louis Joel Feit. According to Dr. Feit, during the sixties, a number of patients who had had hair transplants—"what I call sodding, just as you would sod a lawn"—came to him complaining of honeycomb scars resulting from improperly done transplants. To them, the scars were worse than the original bald spot.

Dr. Feit explains that he began to research the technique and realized that since plugs are a common dermatological method, it made sense for dermatologists to use them to graft skin from one area to another. However, when plastic surgeons had to replace skin lost through an accident or other cause, they would undermine part of the scalp and move it over to the area where it was needed. Often, they noticed that as a result, hair would grow where none had grown before, although this was not the main point of the surgery.

Dr. Feit studied the technique specifically as a means of hair replacement, and he explains in an interview with Rae Lindsay, for her book *How to Look As Young As You Feel* (Pinnacle, 1980), "Basically the principle of the bilobe flap involves undermining the scalp and moving the skin with hair over to the bald area. An incision is made along the margin of the hair so that it will be hidden; the scalp is undercut and replaced. This is a rather extensive procedure, however, and can only be done by an experienced surgeon. The results were quite successful, with the only deterrent a very fine scar line and a rather stalky appearance to the hair, which could be overcome by putting in a few transplanted plugs."

This method of hair replacement also achieves a bit of a face lift, since some skin is pulled up from the face as well as moved over on the scalp.

Dr. Feit's bilobe flap transplant was regarded as an interesting idea but then was discarded by the medical profession in general, and plastic surgeons in particular, until a few years ago, when suddenly the flap technique was identified, in quite separate news announcements, as a "new" procedure perfected by Dr. José Juri of Buenos Aires and by Dr. Ivo Pitanguy, the famous plastic surgeon based in Rio de Janeiro. *The Journal of the American Medical Association,* which had for the most part ignored the studies of Dr. Feit, heralded this "new" technique and reported that one strip, one flap, was equal to about three hundred of the circular plugs transplanted by Dr. Orentreich's method. Moreover, according to the *JAMA* report, while Dr. Orentreich's plugs can only be implanted a few at a time, as many as three flaps can be shifted to balding areas during one procedure. In addition, the flap method produces a denser head of hair in a shorter amount of time than the traditional punch transplant.

Strip Grafting

A variation of the bilobe flap has had limited popularity because doctors and patients alike feel the results look artificial. With strip transplants, two narrow strips of hair from the back or sides of the head are grafted to the forehead to form a new hairline, and then some cosmetic "plugs" are added in front of and behind the grafts. Dr. Arnold Klein, a Los Angeles dermatologist, feels that such stripping produces a very phony hairline, even if a few token "buckshot transplants" are used. Instead, he favors the bilobe flap procedure as a much more realistic approach.

Hair Weaving

A hair-replacement technique less permanent than hair transplant, the bilobe flap, or strip grafting, is called hair weaving, and was invented by black women many years ago. As they say, necessity is the *Mother* of invention. Before the days of Black-Is-Beautiful and the proud presentation of afros, black women believed that straight hair was ideal. To reach this end they would use harsh products (even lye) to straighten the hair. Predictably, often that abused hair responded by falling out. To camouflage the bald areas, black women developed a method of weaving their own hair as the foundation for attaching permanent hairpieces.

When hair weaving is done today, the client's hair is interwoven with nylon cord to form a one-eighth-inch-thick braid long enough to circle the bald spot. This braid is attached to the hair all around the bald spot and then a small hairpiece (usually made of synthetic hair) is attached to the braid. The end result looks quite natural, and one can swim or shower without losing the hair. But keep in mind that your own hair is constantly growing that half-inch per month. This loosens the fit of the piece that's been woven in, and therefore you have to go to a specialist to have that hairpiece tightened about six times a year. The hairpiece itself should be replaced about every three years. It's interesting that most hair-weaving customers are men, even though the technique was originally developed by and for women. But I find hair weaving is a "grasping at straws" remedy and I have reservations about recommending it, as discussed above.

Surgical Implants

A newer, semipermanent technique involves a combination of weaving and surgical implants. Instead of the patient's own hair plugs being used as a replacement, a synthetic hairpiece is chosen. Instead of using a braid to attach the hairpiece, five or six incisions are made in the patient's scalp (usually by a doctor), then a small suture of wire or plastic is made about one-eighth inch below the skin. There's a brief waiting time of four to five hours before a matched hairpiece is permanently sewn to the sutures. The patient returns for a checkup about every twelve months (at this time if any hair has been lost, it's replaced in the hairpiece).

There have been some problems with medical implants caused by infections or by sutures breaking; but today they are using sutures made of O-Prolene (also used for heart surgery) which are not readily rejected by the body.

Dermatologists and doctors still have some reservations about the process, mainly in the area of rejection and infection. Another problem is that if scalp disorders or diseases occur beneath the artificial hairpiece, the whole thing has to be removed to treat them.

Acupuncture

Recently, there have been some interesting advances to alleviate baldness in both men and women via a discipline totally removed from hormone therapy or more traditional forms of hair replacement: acupuncture. Dr. Stanley Du Brin of Van Nuys, California, has been treating victims of hereditary pattern baldness with acupuncture, and in his book *Acupuncture and Your Health,* reported that in several cases patients who formerly had three- or four-inch-wide bald spots had experienced a complete regrowth of hair.

Another physician, Dr. Ryszard Kobos, director of the Aesthetic Surgery Center in Warsaw and president of the Polish Acupuncture Association, reported that of 395 patients (40 of them women), 351 showed excellent hair improvement after acupuncture, 23 had good new hair growth, 14 had satisfactory improvement and only 7 measured no change. Dr. Kobos observed, in a 1976 UPI interview, "Certain acupuncture points have a direct influence on hair growth, and if applied early enough acupuncture will stop hair loss, cause regrowth of hair and make surgical intervention [transplants] unnecessary."

Interestingly, Dr. Kobos also used acupuncture in association with hair transplants and found that when a patient had acupuncture while undergoing transplant surgery, new hair grew back much faster.

Topical or Internal Approaches to Hair Replacement

Despite the general debunking of magic lotions and potions, the hope for hair replacement out of a bottle or via a pill still perseveres. I present some of the latest and ongoing theories to you for the sake of information, urging you as always to take such "miracle remedies" with a grain of salt—perhaps while you're taking your normal array of vitamins.

Megavitamins and Protein Supplements

The late Adelle Davis, a respected nutritionist, thought the answer to hair loss could be found by supplementing inositol intake. In her book *Let's Eat Right to Keep Fit,* she noted, "A few years ago I became interested in the possibility that a lack of inositol [a B vitamin which when deficient in animal diets causes their hair to fall out and when added to their diets again causes their hair to grow back] might be one cause of baldness in men. For a time I recommended inositol together with other sources of B vitamins to all the bald men who consulted me. In almost every case they soon reported that their hair was no longer falling out."

Another nutritionist who has experimented with vitamins and hair regrowth is Dale Alexander. In his book *How I Stopped Growing Bald and Started Growing Hair* he places great faith in his vitamin B-rich Alexander Hair Cocktail, made with milk, raw eggs, wheat germ, wheat germ oil, fruit and sunflower seeds.

Recently, there has been some reported success with another protein—unflavored gelatin. Dr. James Scale, of the Gillette Research Institute in Maryland, gave two groups of people (a total of 103 men and women) 14 grams of unflavored gelatin every day for two months. Hair diameter, which, of course, makes an entire head of hair look fuller and thicker, increased by an average of 9.3 percent in one group and 11.3 percent in the second. Although the increases ranged from 5 to 45 percent, the largest increases occurred in people with the thinnest hair.

Russian Research

Several years ago Russian scientists reported the development of a "magic elixir" to combat baldness. So far, the preparation, called Mival, has been tried on guinea pigs only. According to the Russian journal *Trud,* not only do the guinea pigs grow hair five times normal length, but their offspring were born with much more hair and resembled poodles.

Hungarian Headlines

According to recent headlines in the New York *Times* (April 27, 1980), Hungary has become a center for new theories on hair restoration. Leading the pack, as it were, is a former factory supervisor from Békéscsaba in southeastern Hungary, a man named Andras Banfi, who claims to have invented a miracle cure for regrowing hair. Banfi has studied ancient Egyptian manuscripts and other historical documents and has developed a formula to save his own hair based on his research. After years of study and various formulas, he declares that he has found the solution and saved his hair in the bargain. Now he is marketing his secret, called "Mr. Banfi's Lotion," which has started a rage in Budapest and other areas of Hungary. Although the lotion has a terrible odor and an ugly brownish color (doctors say it consists of alcohol, orange oil, royal jelly from bees and other ingredients), at least one Hungarian dermatological clinic has said the solution might actually help restore hair.

Banfi says the treatment takes six months and requires five bottles of lotion at three dollars a bottle. In my opinion, one of the major ingredients of his potion is that it offers hope, an element that has been included in most hair-replacement remedies for a couple of thousand years. According to the *Times* report, one student, named Laszlo, has been applying the stuff for months with no real results. His father said, "It stinks like garlic. You can't go near him for hours after he puts it on," he noted. "I myself would rather wear a wig."

But Mr. Banfi's Lotion has become a popular remedy for hair restoration and has made its way to Vienna, where it is selling at black-market prices for a hundred dollars a bottle or more.

Another Hungarian, Jeno Nedeczky, from a northern village called Szigethalom, also claims to have developed a remedy for stopping hair loss. Her formula is called "Patientia" because you need a great deal of patience before you see any results. We're still waiting for positive reports.

Aside from Mr. Banfi and Ms. Nedeczky, according to the New York *Times* report, the fight against a receding hairline may become a major Hungarian industry. One hotel manager recently announced a program for foreigners to try to turn the tide of balding, and other managers have joined together to invite tourists to participate in three-day hair-restoring clinical experiments at sixty dollars a day. The offer was taken up by thousands of Germans and other Europeans, and at last count, twelve thousand Greeks had registered for the experiment.

While all this is going on, Andras Banfi, inventor of Mr. Banfi's Lotion, is somewhat distressed. "My friends and everyone made fun of me," he told a New York *Times* reporter. "They said I'm a crazy fool." He was so put off by this adverse reaction that he has dropped work on another pet project—a lotion which would actually *stop* hair growth!

Rumanian Remedies

In Rumania, Dr. Ana Aslan, the octogenarian who discovered Gerovital H-3, and her state-supported clinics have become a tourist attraction and the source of more than a little revenue for this country. Gerovital, a derivative of procaine (yes—the same stuff your dentist shoots you full of when you're getting rid of some current caries), has long been touted as a rejuvenative drug, taken in either pill or injection form. Among the famous patients who have reportedly enjoyed the benefits of Gerovital are the late John F. Kennedy, Chairman Mao, Stalin, Khrushchev, Sukarno, Henry Wallace and Charles de Gaulle, and the still-among-us Marlene Dietrich, Kirk Douglas and Salvador Dalí, plus thousands of others.

While Gerovital is reputed to add fifteen years to one's life and is used for treating depression, smoothing wrinkles, improving memory and concentration, fading out and preventing liver spots, increasing energy and improving skin and muscle tone and sexual drive and performance, another fringe benefit is that it improves the quantity of hair and restores gray hair to former color. Keep in mind though, that Gerovital H-3 has not been approved for use in the United States and that some of its wonder-working properties have never been verified in standard laboratory tests.

American Announcements

Not infrequently, major medical advances come about quite by accident. This was the case when puerperal fever, which sometimes afflicted women who had just had babies, was conquered mainly because doctors washed their hands before delivering babies, and when a crust of moldy bread led to the discovery of penicillin. In this same category, some years ago the Upjohn Company based in Kalamazoo, Michigan, produced a generic drug called minoxidil to assuage and reduce severe high blood pressure. After several years of research, the company's scientists realized that not only does minoxidil reduce hypertension, but it also produces hirsutism in some patients—random and thick hair growth.

Unfortunately, this growth is not limited to bald heads. Some patients who take minoxidil have reported hair growing out of their noses, ears, stomachs, as well as arms and faces. But there is no question that minoxidil produces hair growth. In one study, Dr. Anthony R. Zappocosta of Bryn Mawr, Pennsylvania, reported in *The New England Journal of Medicine* (December 1980) that he had used the drug to treat a patient who had suffered from male pattern baldness for eighteen years. "Within four weeks," the doctor wrote, "dark brown hair grew over the area of the scalp that had previously been devoid of hair visible to the naked eye and had made up the major portion of this scalp except for the sides and the back of the head."

The Upjohn Company, noting the results of these early experiments and research, is now attempting to develop a solution of minoxidil that will stimulate hair growth without lowering blood pressure, and will grow hair where people want it, on their *heads* instead of on or from noses, stomachs, ears, etc.

To that end they have financed investigations by Dr. Howard Baden of the Harvard Medical School and Dr. Norman Orentreich, whose name you know well by now. To date the drug has been tested on about forty inmates of the state prison in Jackson, Michigan, who have voluntarily had their bald heads rubbed with the drug in lotion form.

Even if minoxidil proves to be a reasonable way of restoring hair loss, we're still a few years away from the point when government regulations can be satisfied and pharmaceutical production can be scheduled.

Chapter Ten

The Artful Deceivers

If the procedures mentioned in the last chapter—transplants, bilobe flaps, strip grafting, hair weaving, surgical implants and topical or internal approaches—seem too drastic for you, but you would still like to appear in public with some hair on your head, there is another alternative: a toupee or wig.

I think anyone who opts to replace his hair through temporary means is taking very positive steps toward self-help. No one, male or female, should experience psychological trauma because of the lack of hair. A toupee, commonly known as a "rug," might be the ideal solution.

Selecting a Hairpiece

If a wig or hairpiece is your temporary (but ongoing) solution to your hair-loss problem, there are some points to keep in mind, some rules to follow. If you had very thin hair before, please don't have a very thick hairpiece sitting on it now. It looks artificial, just unbelievably bad. You'll remember that when Bing Crosby wore a toupee you could never tell where his hair ended and his false hair began because there wasn't too much of it and in texture and color it was identical to his own hair. Burt Reynolds also has fine, artfully crafted toupees which look totally realistic.

If you opt for false hair, you should own not one hairpiece or wig but several, so that when you have one or two toupees cleaned and serviced—which you should make a faithful habit so your surrogate hair always looks its best—you'll still maintain your chosen image.

Problems with Toupees

You must realize that hairpieces are very hot and on a really warm day you'll feel as if you're wearing a crash helmet which catches all the heat. Another problem is that wearing the same hairpiece constantly will crossbreed any scalp infections and irritations; in addition, some of the adhesives used to keep a toupee in place can cause allergic reactions in some people. One excellent adhesive remover for toupees and hairpieces that are attached directly to the scalp is Tomae Whisk Adhesive Remover Packet, by American Hospital Supply Company. This product consists of a remover-soaked pad sealed in a little foil packet for freshness. Leading dermatologists recommend it as the safest and best on the market; incidentally, it's also formulated for use in hospitals to remove adhesive tapes used in dressings and bandages.

Another point about wearing wigs and toupees that most people don't realize is that the skin is a water reservoir of the body. As such, it breathes out, never in. And if it doesn't have a chance to breathe out because it's suffocated by extraneous objects (whether wigs, toupees, hats or scarves), any problems you may have had with poor hair growth to begin with are exacerbated. If you wear a wig or hairpiece, always remove it six to ten times a day for about ten minutes so your scalp can breathe.

How to Care for a Hairpiece

While caring for the scalp is always important, you must also learn how to care for your wig or toupee. Here are some hairpiece-care tips, directly from Paul Fleischer of Joseph Fleischer, whose family has been making fine wigs and hairpieces for a hundred years.

1. Before you wash your wig, comb out all teasing or tangles.

2. Fill a little basin with cold water and enough mild shampoo to make suds, or use professional wig cleaner (available in beauty supply stores).

3. Wash the inside of your wig first, using a washcloth dipped in the shampoo solution. Rub off any visible makeup and dirt on the band or around the face.

4. Then immerse the wig in the basin and swish it back and forth for several minutes. Rinse thoroughly in lukewarm water until the water is perfectly clear. All the shampoo must be rinsed out because residue will attract dirt and dust.

5. To dry, squeeze out excess moisture and place wig on a block or stand, preferably one a half-size smaller than your own head size.

6. Comb into place when dry. A good rule of thumb when choosing a wig brush or comb is "Don't use anything on your wig that you wouldn't use on your own hair and scalp." While synthetic pieces will always resume the style programmed into them, with real hairpieces you will have to reset and restyle them.

7. Always store your wig on a block, covered to protect it from dust.

Chapter Eleven

What You Eat Is What You Get

There are some facts of life we all have to learn to live with. For example, if you want to lose weight, you have to eat less or exercise more or both; there's no magic pill, including the faddish "starch blockers," that's going to allow you to eat whatever you want to while you pare off twenty or thirty pounds. Another fact of life we all have to accept is that if you want to be wealthy, with a fat portfolio of blue-chip stocks and investment properties, you'll have to work hard to meet your goal —unless you inherit a fortune or win a million-dollar lottery. Most of us aren't so lucky.

I raise this point because there are facts of life about hair too. If you want a good, healthy head of hair—and I've never met a man who doesn't—you'll never succeed if you don't feed your hair (and your body) with the right combination of nutrients—not just food, but nutrients. Even if you've inherited abundant, thick hair from generations of ancestors (and this is actually money in the bank, so to speak), you'll bankrupt your legacy if you don't nourish and nurture the "property" carefully. Just as a pill can't magically make you lose weight, all the external applications, treatments, products, in the world can't take the place of what you eat. Somebody said, "You are what you eat," and that's true. I prefer, though to say, "What you eat is what you get," and hair is the first reflection of this.

If you play golf, or live in the suburbs, or are a city dweller who visits friends in the country, you'll notice that some lawns are different from other lawns. Here's a green expanse, lush and thick, that you'd like to walk barefoot through. And next to it is a sparse, dried and brown-looking wasteland. The two lawns look so different because they've had different diets: one has been fed and fertilized and watered properly; the other has been neglected and is literally starving for food. It's a good analogy that only breaks down in terms of hair when you consider how a lawn is fed and how your hair is fed. With grass you apply nutrients from the outside in, and they seep into the soil; with hair, the "greening" power is conveyed from the *inside out.*

Remember, though, that since skin which produces hair is the least important of all the human organs, it gets from your blood what is "left over" after the vital organs—the heart, lungs, liver—have had their fill. Therefore, whenever there is a nutritional deficiency the hair, like grass produced by unfertilized soil, is the first to show the effects of this shortage. In this sense, hair is a barometer of health. (In fact, it is a diagnostic factor in spotting such diseases as thyroid deficiencies, which give the hair a very cloudy, limp appearance.)

Unfortunately, most people, men especially, know little about nutrition and care less; after all, it's still women who do most of the cooking and meal planning and have the job of making sure children eat "sensibly." The Basic Four Food Plan is something you learned about in grammar school and conveniently forgot. We are all more interested in having our cake and eating it too, until the waistline expands, and then we want to diet off excess weight in two or three days—instant shape-up.

I've found in all my years of informal research that if I ask what is the most important food, most men and women will say *meat.* But that's absolutely inaccurate. Think of the strongest animals in the world. A bull, for example, or an elephant, a hippopotamus, a cow or a horse. They are all vegetarians, and a good bit healthier than those of us who gorge on meat. They get all the necessary body-building proteins and nutrients from a vegetarian diet.

We humanoids only started eating meat to begin with after discovering that animals "roasted" during forest fires smelled good, and what smelled good tasted good, too. We've been enjoying barbecues ever since. But there was no physical need for meat. Remember that Adam and Eve were evicted from the Garden of Eden because of an apple, not a *steak*.

I'm not suggesting that you should give up meat completely and become a vegetarian, but I have to point out that the people all over the world with the healthiest hair, men and women alike, are those who do not consider meat the most important part of their diets. India, for example, is an undernourished country but the population by and large is blessed with thick and healthy hair. Standard fare is raw or cooked vegetables and meat is a luxury, not a staple, but those who eat adequately (I'm not talking about the poverty-stricken population, although surprisingly many have healthy hair) have enough proteins to maintain energy and good health as well as good skin and hair. Remember, too, they are living on a diet of natural, unprocessed foods. Another example can be found in the Japanese and Chinese people, where again, the diet is made up mainly of vegetables and grains such as rice, with a minimum of "meat," and that mainly in the form of poultry, fish and lean meats. If you try to buy a steak in Tokyo today it will cost about thirty dollars—but then, why bother, when there are so many other, more interesting foods to choose?

In these countries and so many others around the world, meat, poultry and fish are a supplement to the diet, not the main staple. People eat vegetables and salads and fruit and grains predominantly, and meat is added to balance the diet in the same way that most Americans add salad to balance the diet. Sweets, which are part of the American way of life, are usually a rare treat—certainly not an everyday occurrence. This inverse ratio of meat and sweets accounts for most of our country's weight and other nutritionally based problems, which range from bad hair and bad teeth to heart attacks and digestive problems.

I've seen the damages of these nutritional imbalances firsthand.

When I was stationed in Germany, toward the end of World War II and afterward, there was a shortage of the foods we Americans take for granted. Every month, each person had no more than one or two eggs, a quarter of a pound of butter and virtually no meat. (If you read William Styron's moving book *Sophie's Choice,* you'll remember that Sophie was sent to a concentration camp because she was caught smuggling part of a ham for her sick mother; such smuggling went on all over Europe.) The Germans and other Europeans lived mainly on vegetables, fruit and greens. But they had enough of these to maintain good health. The men had broad shoulders and flat stomachs; the women had good skin and luxuriant hair and small waistlines. Today, forty years after the war, and economically thriving, Germans suffer all the weight problems we do—and, not surprisingly, the same nutritional deficiencies.

There's an abundance of food, an overabundance of the *wrong* foods, in fact, and it's hard to push away the plate laden with steak, baked potatoes with sour cream, butter-enriched garlic bread and the rest. There is no question that these enemies to your hair are also the enemies to your health in general.

Not only don't we observe a balanced diet, but as Americans we eat too many overprocessed, refined and devitalized foods—the snack foods and potato chips and candies and endless amounts of sugar-laden soft drinks, the imitations, the fake orange juice and grape juice, the fake bacon and fake bread. Recently I read about a new "high-fiber" bread that costs more, has fewer calories and provides about half the fiber you need every day (along the lines of a current diet fad). This bread is made by a very famous plywood company and they make this bread out of WOOD SHAVINGS! Now, I remember that during the war smart prisoners would eat the bark off trees to provide fiber and nutrition for their bodies—as animals do—but would you tell me why any American today has to eat wood shavings and pay more for it, too?

If you want good bread, and not that moist cotton batting, read the labels and you can find any number of whole-grain breads, at fairly reasonable prices, which will give you the fiber you need. And as a matter of fact, none of the good breads will be made from white flour, which is so refined that it's devoid of most nutritional benefits. (That's why they have to add vitamins and minerals to it—to replace the ones taken out in refining.) No matter what they add, however, they cannot replace the valuable wheat germ and bran which were removed in the milling. And as for other nutrients, did you know it would take twenty-six loaves of unenriched white bread to equal the amount of vitamin B in five little fresh green peas? So don't look for vitamin B in white bread.

White sugar is another villain. It has been estimated that every American eats more than a hundred pounds of white sugar a year (two pounds a week). Can you wonder that, despite fluoridation, tooth decay is on the rise? Excessive amounts of sugar can also lead to nervousness, low blood sugar (hypoglycemia), diabetes, alcoholism, poor digestion, constipation, excessive sebum and other disorders. What sugar actually does is take the place of essential nutrients *without* providing us with any benefits. In other words, sugar supplies "empty" calories. If you have a sweet tooth, eat a piece of fresh fruit or a teaspoon of honey. Learn to drink your coffee with little or no sugar and your tea with honey instead of sugar. Have fresh fruit juice instead of a soda, even if your usual choice is one of those awful-tasting "sugar-free" diet sodas.

And of course, all the additives in foods today add nothing but trouble. Not only do they usually detract from the taste, but they can be harmful as well. The long-range effects of many of these chemicals aren't really known yet, although from time to time some synthetic substance is banned because it has killed two thousand rats in a laboratory. In the meantime, why wait for the lab reports? Today, it's a law that all chemical additives must be listed on labels of packaged foods. Read the labels and try to avoid as many chemicals as you can.

Maybe you think it's a drag to read labels. Maybe you don't even shop for food; that's your wife's job, or your girlfriend's job. But I don't accept that. If you shop for a new car, or a new office copier, or a new lawn mower, you read not only the label but the whole body of information about that car or copier or tool. You want to make sure it's going to run properly. The finest machine you'll ever own is your body, and you can't send it back to the manufacturer if it doesn't work well. You're in charge. Read the labels.

Aside from overabundance and an emphasis on the wrong foods, we also inherit eating habits from our families. It's not so much the tendency to be fat that's inherited, but the *pattern of eating* that leads to fatness. Your mother always told you to clean your plate, and here you are, at thirty-two, still eating every last scrap on your plate, when half of everything would have been more than enough. Your mother is Italian or maybe Jewish and she concentrated more on pasta or potato pancakes and sour cream than she did on fresh fruits or salad. Or maybe your mother is Japanese or Korean and she emphasized fish and undercooked vegetables. Which person do you think is not only slimmer but healthier, and with stronger, better hair?

If you're married or living with someone you may be the victim of your mate's patterns of eating. She wants you to join the "clean plate club" and that plate has been loaded with filling, but not necessarily healthy, food. If that's the case, my friend, you have a problem. If she doesn't get the message by reading this book, you may have to take over the kitchen detail.

There are other patterns of eating, though, that specifically affect businessmen (and businesswomen, too). You're late for a meeting in the morning, so you skip breakfast, then grab a cup of coffee and maybe a danish around 10 A.M. Or maybe have nothing until lunch. Lunch is an important conference with a client, so this involves two martinis or two glasses of wine and the daily special (which happens to be Steak Diane), and you don't want your client to feel like a glutton, so you join him in a Napoleon, or apple pie with ice cream, or maybe the chocolate mousse. Perhaps there's another meeting after five, with a couple of more martinis or glasses of wine and a couple of canapés, and then when you finally get home, you don't want to disappoint your lady, so you have the fried chicken and mashed potatoes and broccoli with cheese sauce, and a little piece of chocolate cake. Or, maybe, if you are missing a lady for the time being, you go home, have another drink or two and grab a TV dinner, or maybe make a quick grilled-cheese sandwich (hold the salad, hold the fruit) and stagger into bed, exhausted.

In both situations (lunch and dinner), you've eaten too much (and probably have drunk too much), and you're exhausted, not only because it's been a grueling day, but also because what you've consumed for those twelve or more hours is not the stuff from which energy is derived. You may not be hungry, but you really haven't fed yourself. No matter how elegant the menu was, or how high the price or quality, actually you've been eating junk food all day.

Energy is actually the measure, because when you're eating properly, no matter how grueling the day, you'll still have the extra reserve to go the next yard. For me a normal workday is usually ten to twelve hours, at least half of these on my feet at my salon, where I'm talking to people who are worried about their hair. I wouldn't dream of starting my day without breakfast. And although I don't drink coffee, I must have a large glass of *chai* (our Russian word for tea) to get me going. I don't add sugar, but sometimes, in the Russian custom, I add a scant teaspoon of strawberry preserves. For lunch I usually have a large salad, and more chai, and for dinner Merci, my wife, will usually prepare fish or poultry, plus salad and one or two fresh vegetables. (I have to add a word about vegetables here. Most Americans cook the hell out of anything that once grew in a garden. If you cook an asparagus and it bends over like spaghetti, throw it away and drink the cooking water, because that's where all the vitamins are now. Vegetables should really say "Crunch"—then they're good. Peas, for example, are murdered if they're cooked for more than four minutes.)

If I have a business appointment for lunch, and I do two or three times a week, I'll enjoy lobster, or mussels, or whichever fresh fish the restaurant is offering, and I will have dessert—fresh strawberries or raspberries or melon or a grapefruit which I prefer whole and then peel and section myself. But I'll usually warn Merci in advance to have a very modest meal that evening because as I've gotten older, I know that I can't eat two "dinners" a day and stay at the weight that suits me best.

Patterns of Eating

Only you can control these. But if you want to be healthy and you want your hair to be healthy, you must develop a new way of eating that will achieve these goals.

Vitamin Power

Vitamins provide the energy, the "fuel," to power the body. Chemically speaking, the alphabetized elements we take for granted were first recognized as crucially important substances by Casimir Funk, a Polish scientist, in 1911. By 1912, he had already published research indicating that "vitamines," as he called them, could correct such diseases as scurvy, pellagra and rickets, which were all shown to be based on nutritional deficiencies. Although it wasn't until 1936 that vitamin C was specifically identified as ascorbic acid, which could prevent scurvy and build up resistance against infections, for more than two hundred years doctors and laymen had recognized a vital connection between the lack of citrus fruits and the prevalence of such diseases.

British sailors always included limes in the ships' stores as long ago as the Napoleonic Wars, and every day the sailors received a mixture of lime juice and their daily ration of rum; that's why they were called "limeys." Amundsen and Peary, when exploring the north and south poles, stocked oranges and lemons in their provisions, and when I was a boy in the 1920s, my parents always gave us orange juice; they knew *something* in citrus fruit helped the body.

Another deficiency, which Casimir Funk never did get to investigate, is very common, although few people have ever heard of the name of the vital vitamin that helps correct this problem. I am talking about gray hair! The appearance of gray hair to any extent (not just a strand here or there) should be equivalent to a burglar alarm that tells you you're being robbed—in this case of a vital nutrient. While most women deal with the alarm by bleaching hair, dyeing it or ignoring it, most men insist that they inherited gray hair and live with it. (Often a full head of gray hair can give a man an image of dignity impossible to achieve with a more youthful appearance, as we mentioned before with Cary Grant or Prince Rainier of Monaco.) Inherited or not, dignified or not, research has indicated that gray hair is actually the result of a vitamin deficiency.

The vitamin lacking is para-aminobenzoic acid, otherwise known as PABA, actually a component of the vitamin B complex. As it is with many medical discoveries (including the surprise development of penicillin), the relationship of PABA to gray hair was revealed quite by accident.

In 1945, when the Russians were liberating concentration-camp prisoners, they found many had nutrition-related tuberculosis and other diseases. Although the Russians themselves didn't have all that much food after the war, they did have vitamins, and they began to give prisoners massive amounts of the B group. Within weeks the doctors noticed that not only was the general condition of the prisoners improving, but for many who were prematurely gray, the hair color began to revert to its normal shade.

In time, this finding was reported in medical journals all over the world, and further research was undertaken in laboratory situations, a much better scientific "battleground" than concentration camps. Within a few years, a distinguished colleague in the field of hair specialization, Dr. Benjamin Sieve, of Boston, was involved in a major study. Of course he had a good field of subjects to work with because at that time many people in Boston were prematurely gray—most likely because of their limited habits of eating. Bostonians followed many of the eating patterns of the Pilgrims of three hundred years ago, a diet which emphasized starches and was deficient in the B vitamins, including PABA. As a side effect of poor diet, there were also some fertility problems, which Dr. Sieve was also treating with vitamin therapy, especially PABA. (Remember, this study took place several decades ago; I am sure that the eating patterns of Bostonians have changed for the better, along with the ever-increasing national awareness of proper nutrition.)

Dr. Sieve experimented for over ten years with seventy-eight thousand patients. In a 1959 report, he concluded that although we *don't* inherit gray hair we *do* inherit the patterns of diet from our families, as we mentioned earlier. And it is this inherited way of eating that accounts for premature grayness. When patients were given about 100 milligrams of PABA per day, taken in 30-milligram doses three times daily, gradually the natural color returned. Dr. Sieve's patients ranged in age from sixteen to seventy-four and had been gray for periods of two to twenty-four years. The first changes in pigmentation after treatment with PABA were noticed in about five weeks. Initially, the hair took on a yellowish cast, or a somewhat darker, dusty gray color. Patients began to notice increased luster and general improvement in the health of their hair.

After the yellow and gray stages, the actual darkening process began to occur, although the length of time this next stage took depended on the general physiological condition of each patient.

Dr. Sieve's experiments provided the thrust for current research and therapy using PABA. The noted endocrinologist and obesity specialist Dr. Neil Solomon, author of several best-selling books on weight control (including, most recently, *Dr. Solomon's Proven Master Plan for Total Body Fitness and Maintenance*), has had dramatic results when treating patients for PABA deficiencies. In a 1980 article in *McCall's,* Dr. Solomon recounts the story of Ruth, nineteen years old, whose black hair was turning gray at an alarming rate. His tests revealed a very low level of PABA: "Even laboratory rats will turn prematurely gray if deprived of PABA," he said. "When PABA is restored, they return to a normal color."

Ruth was prescribed a diet rich in PABA—rice bran and polishings, and brewer's yeast tablets especially. According to Dr. Solomon, although her gray hair didn't turn black, it started growing out black from the roots, and within eleven months, when six inches of new hair had grown in, her hair was once more totally black.

Dr. Solomon has found that a copper deficiency can also produce gray hair prematurely, and for patients who have low levels of copper in their blood he has prescribed molasses with good results. (Of course, molasses is rich in the B vitamins as well as other minerals, including iron.)

The results of these tests with PABA point up the extent to which vitamin deficiencies can affect your hair. Here are the crucial vitamins everyone should include for healthy hair and a healthy body, as established by the Food and Nutrition Board of the National Academy of Sciences–National Research Council:

VITAMIN A: For good vision and healthy skin and hair; essential to epithelial tissues. Vitamin A taken in excessive quantities can be dangerous, however (the Recommended Daily Allowance [RDA] is 5,000 international units; 10,000 units is the suggested therapeutic dosage), and this is definitely not a vitamin for self-medication. Get a doctor's prescription and advice before taking any amount over the 10,000 units included in most therapeutic vitamins.

SOURCES: Butter, eggs, cream, whole milk, cheddar cheese, kidneys, liver, salmon, dark-green leafy vegetables, yellow vegetables, fish-liver oils, tomatoes, apricots and cantaloupe.

VITAMIN B: B represents a whole range of vitamins that are the mainstay of optimum health. B vitamins are often utilized as a key ingredient for skin creams and hair conditioners because they furnish necessary nourishment to the skin. Become friends with these B vitamins:

B_1 (*thiamine*): For the circulatory and nervous systems.

B_2 (*riboflavin*): For building and maintenance of body tissues; helps control the eyes' sensitivity to light.

B_6 (*pyridoxine*): Essential to nervous system, blood vessels and red blood cells. Important for healthy teeth and gums.

B_{12} (*cobalamin*): Important for nervous system; prevents certain forms of anemia.

Niacin (*niacinamide*): Prevents pellagra and is essential for converting food into energy. Aids nervous system and stimulates healthy appetite.

Folic acid: Essential for protection of gastrointestinal tract.

Pantothenic acid: For nervous system and adrenal glands and for the manufacture of antibodies.

Biotin: For health of skin and mucous membranes; necessary for maintenance of red blood cells and circulatory system. Biotin is crucial for the production of *E. coli* (*Escherichia coli*)—tiny microorganisms manufactured in the intestines and an essential aid to digestion. (Unfortunately, when antibiotics are prescribed to kill infections, the *E. coli* are also killed by the hundreds of millions. If you have been taking antibiotics, be sure to eat at least one cup of yogurt every day for about a week to maintain the *E. coli*).

PABA (*para-aminobenzoic acid*): In addition to preventing gray hair or restoring natural color, PABA has also been found to be helpful in treating certain skin diseases, such as vitiligo and eczema.

SOURCES: There is a wide selection of foods that supply all of the B's, so you can take your choice and make sure you're getting enough of these vital nutrients—milk, eggs, whole-grain cereals and breads, fish, poultry, beef, pork, lamb, veal, liver and other organ meats, dried yeast, peanuts, nuts and nut butters, oysters, dark-green leafy vegetables, soybeans, molasses, beans, corn.

VITAMIN C: Some experts say that if you can take only one vitamin, this is it! Vitamin C keeps all systems revved up, prevents scurvy, is essential to strength of body cells and blood vessels, and important for healthy teeth, gums and bones.

SOURCES: The highest C content is found in black currant berries; second highest source is horseradish, followed by green peppers and rose hips, and then the citrus fruits as well as strawberries, tomatoes, pineapples, bananas, avocados, artichokes, dark-green leafy vegetables, cabbage and cauliflower.

C is a very fragile and short-lived vitamin, however. If you decide to be efficient and healthy and squeeze a dozen oranges the night before so you and your family can enjoy fresh orange juice for breakfast, you're making a mistake. The taste of fresh juice will still be there, but most of the vitamin C will have disappeared; the life span of fresh C is about four minutes. You're better off with carton-packed "fresh" or frozen O.J. to which they've added ascorbic acid. If you want the "real thing," squeeze the juice when you're ready to drink it.

VITAMIN D: Prevents rickets, helps grow strong teeth and bones, is vital in the process of utilizing calcium and phosphorus.

SOURCES: The sun, especially during warm weather, generates vitamin D; also fish-liver oils, fortified milk.

VITAMIN E (*tocopherol*): This vitamin has a lot of potential that has not yet been proven. It's interesting to me, though, that some of the nation's top gerontologists, who are exploring many different approaches to longevity, routinely take 400 international units of E each day. Whether or not E proves to be the wonder vitamin of the late twentieth century (it's also been touted as a solution to sex problems and heart conditions), we still need vitamin E for good skin and hair as well as to protect fat within the body tissues and control the rate of its breakdown, a process essential for red blood cells.

SOURCES: Unrefined or cold-pressed vegetable oils, fresh or vacuum-packed wheat germ, freshly ground whole-grain breads and cereal.

VITAMIN K: Helps blood clotting.

SOURCES: Most of the body's supply is manufactured by microorganisms in the intestines, but it can also be found in dark-green leafy vegetables, tomatoes, soybeans, liver.

Minerals—Coworkers of Vitamins

Minerals work along with vitamins to help your body function smoothly. Although we actually need about eighteen different minerals, many are provided in adequate amounts with even the poorest diet. Some minerals, however, require special attention:

CALCIUM: For strong teeth and bones, blood clotting, and nerve and muscle activity.

SOURCES: Milk, cheese, dairy products, green vegetables. You also get a small amount of calcium if your normal water supply is hard water.

PHOSPHORUS: Calcium and phosphorus work in chemical combination with each other; if one is missing, the other has nothing to combine with and is wasted. For example, if a person doesn't drink milk or eat other calcium-rich foods, the body dumps phosphorus in the urine without getting its benefits. With a phosphorus deficiency bones break easily and teeth decay.

SOURCES: Dairy products, all foods made from grain, fresh vegetables, meats.

SODIUM: This mineral is truly essential for life, but most of us have to cut down on, not increase, our intake, especially if high blood pressure is a problem. Less salt means less water retention. When people go on major diets what they lose first is excess water because most sensible diet regimens stress little or no salt intake. So initially dieters are losing water, not pounds. In some cases water retention is desired. During the Napoleonic Wars, for example, wounded soldiers were given salted herring and other high-salt-content foods because the resulting edema (or swelling) reduced pain and was good protection against excessive bleeding during surgery.

SOURCES: Common table salt, almost all foods, and present in *soft* water.

IODINE: Iodine is part of thyroxine, the hormone that determines the bodily chemical processes which produce energy from foods. An iodine deficiency can cause poor health, thinning hair, goiter or other serious medical problems.

SOURCES: Ordinary iodized table salt, seafood, kelp.

SULFUR: Absolutely essential for good hair growth (in fact, part of the chemical content of the hair is sulfur).

SOURCES: Can only be obtained from high-quality protein, as described below or in water with a high sulfur content.

IRON: Helps to build good strong blood.

SOURCES: Egg yolks, whole-grain breads and cereals, dried fruit, liver, meat, dried peas and beans, and dark-green leafy vegetables. Although Popeye didn't eat spinach for nothing, if he wanted superstrength he might have been better off eating *grass,* which has a hundred times more nutritional value. Grass is hard to digest, however, and the animals which thrive on it—cows, horses, other grazing breeds —have longer intestines than humans. So in the meantime we'll have to settle for spinach plus the other iron-rich foods listed to provide this very important mineral.

POTASSIUM: For healthy nerves and muscles.

SOURCES: Although small amounts are present in milk, coffee, fish and meat, the very best sources are vegetables, citrus fruits, cantaloupe, bananas and apricots.

ZINC: For the formation of healthy cells. Zinc deficiencies inhibit the production of RNA and DNA (see Nucleic acids, below); adequate zinc is essential for the synthesis of body protein and the action of many enzymes. An undersupply can cause hair problems, diminished fertility, poor resistance to infections and skin abnormalities.

SOURCES: The best natural source known is shellfish; also found in eggs, liver, oysters, herring, seaweed and maple syrup.

Proteins—The Body's Building Blocks

"High protein" has become a common nutritional term, recognized by health-food aficionados and casual eaters alike as a very important quality in food. What few people realize, however, is that all body cells —including hair, of course—contain protein.

Whenever the body suffers from a deficit of protein, drastic changes and malfunctions occur, but one of the first areas to demonstrate this disaster visually is the hair. Some years ago when Biafra was in the news, who could ignore the terrible condition of the starving children with bloated bellies? They were suffering from *kwashiorkor,* a protein deficiency, in which the first symptom is discoloration of the hair: although the children were black, they all had light red hair, an indication of advanced malnutrition.

Since protein is probably the most important nutrient of all, we should know a little about its composition and the chemical characteristics that make it so vital for human health. Protein is composed of carbon, oxygen, nitrogen and hydrogen, plus some minerals. Basically, proteins are combinations of smaller molecules called amino acids, and it is the presence of certain amino acids which makes one protein food more valuable than another.

Although more than twenty-five amino acids have been isolated in proteins, for our purposes it's only necessary to talk about them in general. Amino acids are divided into two groups: *essential* and *nonessential*. Essential amino acids are so called because the body can't produce them; we must get them through the food we eat. Nonessential amino acids, happily, are synthesized from the essential acids. Any food that can provide all the essential amino acids is known as a *complete protein*. Two specific amino acids play significant roles in hair growth: *methionine* (an essential) and *cystine,* which will be produced if an adequate amount of complete protein is included in our diets.

Actually, all natural foods contain some amount of protein. In other words, it's not the *quantity* of protein that you take in every day, but the *quality*. This is one reason why I'm skeptical about the current fad for counting protein grams. The only way to ensure the most beneficial balance of amino acids is to include as much *high-quality* protein in your diet as possible.

Nucleic Acids

High-quality protein is also the best source for increasing the output of cell-building nutrients that have received a great deal of attention recently—nucleic acids. The biological role of these acids has only been discovered within the past twenty-five years. While cells are made up of various types of nucleic acids, the most important are RNA (ribonucleic acid) and DNA (deoxyribonucleic acid), which work together. According to Dr. Benjamin Frank of New York City, who has done extensive research on cells and why they stop functioning, aging is "the deterioration of individual cells . . . to make cells healthy again, we have to provide the substances that nourish and repair them most directly."

With an increased supply of such foods as fish, liver, beets and other vegetables, Dr. Frank's patients have not only regained cellular energy but report feeling better and looking younger. And within three or four months on a nucleic acid-building diet, skin and hair also look healthier. While this is only the briefest view of what has been termed a "no-aging diet," if you concentrate on the proteins we outline for you below, you will guarantee the production of amino acids, nucleic acids and other cell revitalizers.

The Superproteins

Scientists and nutritionists have established a frame of reference for assessing which protein foods are better than others. The term is *biological value,* and the basis is the amount of food required to meet human needs. The less protein required, the higher the biological value. And the food with the highest biological value of all is *the egg.*

The Egg Comes First

The ubiquitous, fragile, inexpensive and artfully shaped egg has the greatest ability to support life—gram for gram—and the largest proportion of the amino acid methionine than any other complete proteins.

Unfortunately, many men limit their egg intake drastically because of the ongoing cholesterol scare. But, in my opinion, this doesn't make sense because eggs contain substantial amounts of lecithin, inositol and choline, three nutrients which battle *against* the collection of cholesterol in the bloodstream.

In addition, eggs contain large quantities (again gram for gram) of vitamins A, B_1, niacin, D and E and many minerals, including sulfur. One raw egg a day can give a real boost to your hair. If you can't take the idea of a raw egg straight, try blending it with milk, fruit and wheat germ for a revitalizing meal in a glass.

For centuries there have been many folk and medical therapeutic cures for various illnesses which relied on the use of eggs. One recipe, for example, used in Russia to combat tuberculosis and in France as a remedy for malnutrition, is still effective today if you have extreme hair fallout caused by prolonged illness or poor eating habits or extended negligence. For a revitalizing booster, break 10 eggs (shells and all) into a large glass bowl; squeeze in the juice of 10 lemons and add 1 cup of raw sugar. Mix well until the eggs are scrambled and the sugar is dissolved, then let it sit at room temperature a day or so until it turns into a pasty-looking liquid. Strain and refrigerate; drink a 4-ounce glass daily.

One of my favorite superprotein recipes using raw eggs always acts as an energy builder and pick-me-up when I'm going through a great deal of stress in my business, or when I'm battling the flu or another debilitating illness. It's a Russian concoction called a "Gogol-Mogol." Here's the recipe: whip 2 eggs yolks with 2 teaspoons of raw sugar in a blender (about ½ cup yield) and eat with a spoon like custard.

Two other ways to use raw egg in a drink, either for a breakfast pick-me-up, or anytime when you need an energy boost include: an eggnog made with beer (8 ounces of beer blended with 1 or 2 whole eggs), or a Marsala eggnog (4 ounces of Marsala blended with 1 or 2 whole eggs, topped with a little cream and a dash of cinnamon).

If the raw-egg route doesn't sit well with you, soft-boiled, hardboiled, scrambled, omelet, or even the old favorite sunny-side-up version will also give you the benefits of this wonderful food.

Make It Milk

If you think milk is for kids, it's time to think again. Milk is a food everybody needs, all their lives. (It's been proven that so many elderly people suffer broken hips and brittle bones mainly because they don't include enough calcium in their diets. All adults should have at least one serving of milk a day, and another serving of a dairy product such as cottage cheese, ice cream or yogurt.)

In this book we're concerned about milk as another complete protein, with built-in extra vitamins and minerals that can spell the difference between healthy hair and sparse, drab-looking hair that looks best hidden under a hat.

While the best milk of all is raw certified milk, this is not readily available (you have to buy it in health-food stores) and is rather expensive. Powdered skim milk, which could be called a convenience food, is ironically, not only inexpensive but retains nearly all the original nutritional values of raw milk. Mix according to directions and use on cereal, or drink it straight. If you have a cooperative lady on hand, have her substitute powdered milk for whole milk in soups, sauces and desserts—she'll benefit, too.

Eat Meat

It's true that many healthy people and most animals in this world never eat meat, but this food should not be disregarded: in certain forms it represents another complete protein. But what we're talking about is *lean* meat—not hot dogs or commercially prepared hamburgers with preservatives, cereals, chemicals and an abundance of bad-for-you fat. Although they may taste good to you, make it a point to limit pork, bacon, ham, sausages, pastrami, beautifully marbled (and fatty) steaks and roasts. The lean meats will not only provide adequate amounts of protein, but they are an excellent source of iron, the B vitamins and other essential vitamins and minerals.

At this point I'd like to comment about faddists who preach the value of eating raw meat, especially in such dishes as steak tartare, and the newest member of the raw meat family, *filetto Carpaccio,* a sliced raw beef dish served with either a mayonnaise- or mustard-based sauce. These dishes may appeal to some people's taste buds, but I'm afraid I must disagree with the health-food cultists who say that raw meat is "live" food. It is not live; it is simply not cooked.

Perhaps the urge for undercooked meat began with sailors centuries ago. When they went to sea, meat spoiled easily in the days before refrigeration and the "cookies," or chefs, after scraping the worms off the meat, would load it with salt or spices and cook it until it was almost burned to disguise the near-rotten condition. When sailors returned home they wanted to eat meat as raw, as fresh, as possible.

Still, we're not cannibals, and meat that has been cooked properly (as opposed to very rare or raw) is easier to digest and produces less uric acid in the system, which helps you avoid the uncomfortable disease known as gout.

For Liver Lovers

People either love liver or hate liver; there's no in-between attitude about this food, which happens to be the most nutritionally complete natural food of all. If you want to build power, strength and a superhealthy body, eat liver—it is the most potent single source of natural blood and body building essentials. Liver also satisfies most body needs for iron, calcium, phosphorus, iodine, copper and other minerals and is rich in vitamins A, B complex and C. And liver is a veritable gold mine for protein.

It wouldn't be very realistic for me to suggest you eat liver every day (even the most enthusiastic liver-eaters could not quite follow this schedule), but there is an alternative: desiccated liver, available in either tablet or powdered form, which, although slightly less nutritious than the real thing, can provide a major proportion of your daily protein needs.

Fish Facts

Fish is another good source of complete protein, an easily digested food, especially favored by weight watchers. If you consider all the areas of the world where fish is, in fact, the nutritional mainstay, you'll see that the people who live in these places have few, if any, hair problems. Among other essential vitamins and minerals, fish is high in iodine, trace minerals and unsaturated fat—a boon for those who might be worried about heart disease.

First Health Food—Yogurt

Maybe you think yogurt is for women who are trying to diet, but, ironically, this nutritious form of milk was discovered thousands of years ago by males—food hunters who set off on long journeys in search of supplies for their families and tribes, equipped with a saddlebagful of milk, which spoiled rather quickly. When you're hungry you eat anything, and what these nomads ate did not taste half bad. In fact, when "doctored up" with spices or fruit or vegetables, it became a nutritious and tasty mainstay. Yogurt is actually a form of fermented milk or lactic acid, and it contains all the nutrients and protein of milk in a form easily assimilated by most people. (The protein has already been broken down and therefore it is very easy to digest.)

We've all heard about the Hunzas in the Himalayas, and the Georgians in Russia who attribute their long lives in part to daily doses of yogurt, and nobody has proved them wrong yet. In the formulation of yogurt, large amounts of the B-complex vitamins are produced, along with "friendly bacteria" which aid digestion and elimination, another key factor for good-looking skin and hair.

The best yogurt is plain, because so many of the "attractive" commercial varieties with fruit added also include sugar and preservatives. It's better to add your own fresh fruit to plain yogurt, but I'm also happy to see that more and more yogurt companies are leaving out the preservatives and refined sugar and producing flavored yogurts which are appealing and healthy. Remember, though, to read the label before you buy.

Here are some of the ways I enjoy yogurt the most: as a substitute for anything that calls for sour cream—try a baked potato topped with yogurt mixed with chives and Worcestershire sauce, plus a dash of lemon juice; or a dollop of yogurt, plus dill with cold borsht or cold tomato soup. I add a couple of tablespoons of yogurt to scrambled eggs, plus some herbs for an elegant but filling brunch or lunch dish. I stir half a cup of yogurt into beef stew for an ersatz and low-calorie "beef Stroganoff." And any time of the year I mix plain yogurt with lemon juice or vinegar, plus chives, dill or oregano as a salad dressing for sliced tomatoes or cucumbers.

One of the most unusual and enjoyable uses for yogurt I've found is a favorite Armenian recipe for a summer beverage. It's called *tahn*. Mix 1 pint of plain yogurt with 1 quart of water and stir well. Pour into an ice-filled glass and enjoy a refreshing pickup on a hot, humid day.

A Salad to Complement any Chicken

You can serve this salad with any style chicken—fried, boiled, broiled, baked. . . . It is my wife's favorite salad and it may become yours as well.

½ bunch scallions
1 teaspoon salt
1 medium cucumber, peeled and sliced
½ bunch radishes
2 heads Boston lettuce
4 ounces sour cream
4 teaspoons sugar
1 8-ounce container plain yogurt

Cut scallions in ½-inch pieces and add salt. Mash lightly with a fork. Add cucumber, mix well and let it bleed. Slice radishes and add for color. Break Boston lettuce into bite-sized pieces and add to salad. Mix in the sour cream until ingredients are well coated. Add sugar to the yogurt and mix lightly. Add yogurt to salad and toss gently. Serve immediately or it will curdle. Serves 4.

Sunflower Seeds

If you're looking for a low-calorie, high-value between-meals snack, stock up on sunflower seeds, a good source of complete protein, high in polyunsaturated fatty acids and a rich mine of vitamins and minerals.

Sunflower seeds are heavily loaded with methionine, the amino acid we've talked about before.

If your store of sunflower seeds gets a little soggy and tastes somewhat blah, put them in a frying pan and brown them very slightly while you shake the frying pan over low heat.

Brewer's Yeast

This is another trendy "health" food, but it deserves its popularity because brewer's yeast is a tremendous source of protein and all the B's. Brewer's yeast is actually a tiny plant, packed with 17 different vitamins, 14 minerals and 16 amino acids. Further, the composition of the yeast cell is very similar to the composition of the cells that make up the human body—a most compatible relationship.

Purists take brewer's yeast in powdered form and mix 2 or 3 tablespoons in soup, health drinks, mashed potatoes, meatloaf and other foods. (It comes in a debittered form which is almost tasteless.) For those who like to swallow their nutrients in "disguised" versions, liquid brewer's yeast is excellent. A total of 100 grams (3½ fluid ounces or 2 tablets) once a day provides about 75 percent of daily protein needs.

High-Protein Supplements

I don't think anyone should take high-protein supplements while dieting, unless under a doctor's care. I'll be talking about diets a little later on, but it's important to say a few words here about these products, which have become a popular diet fad in recent years. When these protein supplements (which contain all the essential amino acids, as well as egg albumen, whole and defatted dried milk solids and whole and defatted soy powder) are used as the *only* food substance included in a diet, there have been dangerous side effects and even deaths from the extreme protein intake. Concentrate on the superprotein foods, and when used appropriately one can lose weight and still be healthy, which is the name of the game.

Carbohydrates Add Up to Energy

Carbohydrates have become a dirty word in nutrition, because in our think-thin society, we're too eager to believe that it's bread and rice and noodles that make us fat. To a certain extent that's true, but only when the intake is excessive. Everybody needs some carbohydrates every day because they provide about half of our daily energy requirements. In addition, such a humble food as the potato can contribute a great deal to how your hair looks and grows. Often, it's not the bread, or the rice, or the noodles, or the potatoes that add to weight—it's what we put on them. But if you can't stay away from bread laced with butter or French fried potatoes, you can get your energy requirements and keep your weight down by including high-carbohydrate fruits and vegetables, another excellent, good-for-you source.

There Are Fats and There Are Fats

Fats provide about twice as much energy as an equal amount of carbohydrates, plus we need them to pad the vital organs and help us gain protection from extremes of temperature. Fats also nourish hair and skin cells. Think of the beautiful fur worn by seals and minks, animals which produce fatty oils in abundance.

There are two kinds of fats: *saturated,* basically animal fats—lard, chicken fat, butter, the fat in meats and whole milk; and *unsaturated* fats, obtained from sunflower, olive, soy, corn and cottonseed oils.

How Much of What

Basically then, for the best-looking body and hair you need a balanced supply of protein, carbohydrates, fats, vitamins and minerals. The absence or deficiency of any of these in your diet will have a very visible and drastic effect on how you look and feel. And it's preferable that you obtain most of these substances from natural food which you eat. Although there are some instances where vitamin supplements are indicated, always keep in mind that pill-popping can't really take the place of eating the right foods. And vitamin pills give you no esthetic sense of eating pleasure, either. Isn't it nicer to eat an orange than to take 100 milligrams of vitamin C?

You should try to work your daily eating around the Basic Four Plan, which includes all the nutritional requirements we've discussed. And if you follow the moderate but adequate portions suggested, you won't starve, nor will you gain weight.

MILK: Two servings daily—one or two glasses of whole, skim, evaporated, dry or buttermilk. An ounce of cheese, one serving of ice cream, half a pint of yogurt, each counts as one serving of milk.

VEGETABLES AND FRUIT: Four or more servings daily—one should be citrus or tomato (for vitamin C); at least four times a week include a dark-green or deep-yellow vegetable or fruit for vitamin A; at least once a week dried fruit or dried beans for extra protein and iron.

MEAT: Three servings daily—beef, veal, other lean meats, liver, poultry, fish or eggs, for protein, iron, vitamins and necessary fat; at least one lunch-sized serving (an egg or an ounce of cheese, meat or canned fish); one dinner-sized serving, 2 or 3 ounces of meat, fish or poultry.

BREAD AND CEREALS: Four servings daily to provide carbohydrates, vitamins and minerals. Preferably whole grain, nonrefined. One serving equals a slice of bread, or ¾ cup of "dry" cereal, or ½ cup of cooked cereal, cornmeal, macaroni, noodles or rice.

Why Water and Other Liquids?

In addition to all the nutrients we've been talking about, everybody needs from 6 to 8 glasses of liquid a day to help keep a good supply of liquid circulation in the body and encourage regular elimination. Remember, too, that skin is the reservoir of water, so it must be replenished, in the same way that we water our plants to replace lost moisture. Every day we lose about 4½ pints of water through perspiration and elimination. To replace this amount, it doesn't require that you run out and drink 8 glasses of water a day; while water is good for you, soup and juice and coffee count, too.

And Now the Big Question of Fiber

Fiber used to be called roughage, but perhaps the new name is more glamorous. Call it whatever you want, fiber or roughage is the best way to prevent constipation—the worst enemy of any sensible nutritional program. Some of the most common symptoms of constipation are lack of appetite, nervousness and listlessness. Constipation also affects the digestion and proper assimilation of all the nutrients we've discussed; it actually short-circuits the process of regeneration of the cells that build strong tissues. One of the main causes of constipation today is the use of refined white sugar and flour, which discourages elimination of wastes and toxins, a process necessary for good health. To correct this, concentrate on foods high in fiber (whole grains and cereals, for example, especially bran), fresh fruit and vegetables and nuts.

Another fiber attracting attention today is *pectin,* the substance that makes jelly gel and is found in the inner rind of citrus fruits. According to Dr. Alastair Connell, of the University of Cincinnati, "The data available suggest that the pectins are the most valuable single group of fibers because they absorb bile salts and cholesterol, so the excretion of cholesterol is increased." In a recent article in *Harper's Bazaar,* Dr. Connell suggested that the best way to get pectin is by eating apples and pears with the skins on or by eating the white part of oranges and grapefruits.

The Right Diet Pares Weight, Builds Energy

Today we live in a hi-tech age where electronic and other miracles occur as fast as you can snap two fingers together. The expectation of instant results carries through even with something as tricky as dieting. We forget that those extra pounds weren't gained in a day or a week. All we can think about is how fast we can lose them. Unfortunately, not only can crash diets do a great deal of harm, but they are tremendously unpleasant to experience. According to Dr. Lawrence E. Lamb, who writes a daily nationally syndicated newspaper column on health and medicine, "Crash diets can cause fatigue. If you are on one of those widely publicized low-carbohydrate diets, or worse, one with almost no carbohydrates, you will feel tired. The absence of carbohydrates in your diet causes your kidneys to flush out sodium and water." In an article in *Harper's Bazaar,* he wrote, "This loss makes a dramatic change in the number of pounds that show on the scales, but it does not eliminate fat. It dehydrates you and upsets your body chemistry."

In addition, when you cut out most foods with a crash diet, you change your hormonal balance and these important messengers (for that is the function of hormones) are actually *shocked.* In turn this produces shocking results to your hair and other body systems.

If you must diet, do it sensibly and slowly with an aim of losing no more than three or four pounds a week, and above all, avoid faddish one-food diets. My work takes me all over the world, and often my hosts in other cities and countries feel obliged to entertain me in the grand style. I can't refuse to participate in their gala dinners without appearing rude. You don't tell someone who has arranged a magnificent banquet ranging from caviar to Scottish salmon to the whitest veal possible to the most exquisite pastries ever devised that you are "on a diet." Consequently, sometimes I gain five or ten pounds over my normal weight of 180. When that happens I immediately begin my "Easy-Does-It Diet," which has provided excellent results for me and dozens of my friends for years.

This is a diet plan that is especially healthful for men because it eliminates fat without affecting muscle tone. All you have to do is set a goal of how much weight you want to lose, and if the amount is anything over fifteen pounds, or if you have a heart ailment or any hereditary problems, you must consult a doctor first. The rules are strict, but if you follow them you'll enjoy the rewards. There are six don'ts:

No sugar or sugar substitutes
No salt or salt substitutes
No soups
No alcohol, including wine and beer
No juice of any kind
No melon of any kind

My plan is not a diet for better or worse. I like to think it's better . . . and it works. Here's how: you must have six meals a day—not one or three or two but *six,* and you must drop all strenuous exercise for the time being. Instead, walk; walk about five miles a day at a normal pace, preferably one hour before bed. Each meal must be scheduled at three-hour intervals, and the most important meal is breakfast (as it is for people who aren't dieting). The following schedule is for my day which begins at eight. Tailor it to your own time plan.

BREAKFAST: 8 A.M.
   1 fruit (if you like grapefruit, eat it like an orange)
   1 egg, soft boiled, or
   2 slices of bacon, crisp, or
   2 Jones breakfast sausages, crisp
   ½ slice whole-grain bread, toasted or plain
   1 teaspoon butter
   Hot tea (preferred to coffee), no lemon or sugar

MIDMORNING: 11 A.M.
   3 teaspoons powdered skim milk in 4 ounces water
   1 ounce Swiss Emmenthaler or Jarlsberg cheese

LUNCH: 2 P.M.
   ½ head lettuce
   1 3-ounce can tuna or salmon, without oil
   1 teaspoon sunflower-seed oil
   Mix as a salad and sprinkle with lemon juice
   Tea

MIDAFTERNOON: 5 P.M.
   Powered skim milk and cheese, as at 11 A.M.

DINNER: 8 P.M.
   1 6-ounce shell steak or
   1 small fish, or
   1 lamb chop, or
   1 pork chop (any of these must be lean and broiled)
   1 baked potato; eat either the pulp or the skin; if you want to eat both, then eat only ½ potato, or
   1 stalk broccoli or cauliflower (avoid peas, dried beans and carrots)
   ⅓ head lettuce plus 2 slices tomato or *2 radishes* or *2 strips green or red pepper, dressed with sunflower-seed oil and sprinkling of lemon juice*

1 piece fruit, preferably the hybrid type such as nectarines or
tangelos

LATE EVENING: 11 P.M. (AFTER WALKING AND BEFORE BED)
3 teaspoons powered milk in 4 ounces water
1 generous teaspoon peanut butter

I'm not going to tell you you're not going to miss having a drink or a piece of cake or candy the first two days. But if you can curb your emotions and your appetite for forty-eight hours you'll adapt to this regimen very smoothly and within one week you'll forget that sugar and salt taste very different from each other.

Ideally, on this plan, the first week you'll lose four pounds, the second week three pounds and the third and following weeks, three or four pounds. But what you'll be losing is fat, not muscle. You should supplement this, and most other diets, with a multiple vitamin (taken after breakfast), plus 1900 milligrams (19 grams) lecithin and 400 units of vitamin E; and up to 15 tablets a day of natural vitamin C, 100-milligram strength, taken throughout the day and not at once.

Of course, the best approach is to maintain your ideal weight all the time. Often the yo-yo syndrome produced by going on and off diets creates hair problems that could have been avoided, not to mention what it does to the elasticity of your skin. How many times do you expect to stretch six or seven inches across the stomach, lose twenty pounds and have that skin and muscle tone snap back? It only happens two or three times.

By now you know how to eat your way to healthy hair—and you've also learned something about my own eating preferences as well. A Johns Hopkins doctor once told me, "Eat anything that will rot, but eat it before it rots." The major point is that I don't eat things that can "eat" me. I eat very little meat (perhaps only once a month) and fruit and vegetables all the time. My main diet is fish and seafood, plus undercooked or steamed vegetables, fresh fruit and usually cheese for dessert. But my favorite food of all is a magnificent salad, made with twenty ingredients and as appetizing to look at as it is good for you.

Aside from the array of vegetables as fresh as I can find them, the secret of my salad is sunflower-seed oil. This oil comes from the flower that actually turns with the sun, and it is laden with vitamin E and other nutrients. Don't make the mistake of buying *unrefined* sunflower oil, however. The refined version is just as healthful and better-tasting, and in your salad it will coat each vegetable tenderly, unlike olive oil, which has a tendency to overwhelm a lettuce leaf. (Always store unused sunflower-seed oil in the refrigerator.)

My Favorite Salad Recipe

½ bunch scallions, green and white parts, cut in ½-inch pieces
Salt (about 1 teaspoon)
½ small white onion, sliced
½ Bermuda onion, sliced
1 bunch radishes, sliced
1 cucumber, peeled and sliced
1 green pepper, seeded and diced
1 carrot, cut in ¼-inch slices
2 stalks celery, cut in chunks
¼ pound raw green peas, shelled
½ head Boston lettuce, torn in bite-sized shreds
½ head regular or iceberg lettuce, torn in bite-sized shreds
⅓ bunch watercress, coarsely chopped
2 lemons
2 Belgian endives, halved and then sliced
⅓ cup sunflower-seed oil
¼ pound fresh mushrooms, sliced
2 ripe tomatoes, quartered
1 ripe avocado, sliced
Pepper to taste
½ cup fresh dill, cut in ½-inch pieces

1. Drop the scallions into a large salad bowl and sprinkle with salt. Then, with a fork, "bleed" the scallions, mashing them until they are fairly limp.

2. Next, add the white and Bermuda onion slices, and the radishes. Toss well (every time you add a new ingredient, toss the salad). Add the cucumber, green pepper, carrots, celery and peas. Toss in the lettuce and watercress, and gently mix all ingredients.

3. Cut the lemons in half and squeeze the juice over the salad. Add the endives and then sprinkle the sunflower-seed oil over the salad. Mix well. Gently stir in the mushrooms, tomatoes and avocado slices. Add pepper. Taste for seasoning.

4. Finally, add the fresh dill. Let the salad sit for five minutes before serving.

This is a very generous salad for four, and if you have leftovers they'll keep for a day or two in a plastic container in the refrigerator. Don't be put off by wilted lettuce; actually the salad tastes even better the next day. If you're under dental care and have problems chewing, put the whole salad in a blender and then drink it—delicious!

Epilogue

I'm happy to have written this book as a companion piece to my earlier work, *George Michael's Secrets for Beautiful Hair* (Doubleday, 1981), because what began as a hobby many years ago—my interest in healthy, shining hair—has turned into my life's dedication. For the past quarter of a century, I've been collecting material for both books, and after all this time, I realize that three important elements went into the writing of them: a tremendous amount of education, a tremendous amount of practical experience and certainly, not least of all, a tremendous amount of love.

Although these books have been my dream for decades, it was always a dilemma to find the time to write. My office at my busy Madison Avenue salon in New York was not a haven because of the constant interruptions and personal consultations with clients who travel from all parts of the world to see me. Ultimately, I found the time and energy to write as I traveled in Europe, Asia, England, the Caribbean, South America and the United States for both business and pleasure. (Today over sixty salons in Belgium, Germany, Great Britain and Switzerland are affiliated with me and follow my doctrine for sensible, effective hair care.) Because so much of my writing has been done in other parts of the world, I would like to share with you the list of marvelous locations—some tranquil, some stimulating—that played a great role in inspiring my work.

The Islands:

St. Thomas (Morningstar Beach resort, where I always stay) and St. John (Caneel Bay) in the American Virgin Islands, Antigua, Jamaica, Puerto Rico, Virgin Gorda's Little Dix Bay and Dr. Ivan Popov's famous Renaissance Spa in Nassau, the Bahamas.

Far East:

Bali (Partamina Cottages), Djakarta (Hilton Hotel), Indonesia; Republic of Singapore (Goodwood Park Hotel, Mandarine Hotel), Hong Kong (Regent Hotel).

The International Cities:

Rome, Paris (Intercontinental Hotel and Hôtel Meurice), London (Park Tower and Claridge's Hotel), Zürich (Zum Storchen), Gottlieben (Hotel Krone), San Remo (an Italian gem), and the French Riviera.

American Cities:

San Francisco (Fairmont Hotel), New Orleans (Roosevelt Hotel), Miami Beach (Golden Strand Hotel and Villas), Honolulu (Hilton Hawaiian Village, Waikiki Beach).

Ski Resorts:

Franconia, New Hampshire, and Mittersille on Cannon Mountain, New Hampshire; Stowe, Vermont (Topnotch); The Berkshires (Jugend Resort); Montreal (Holiday Inn Chateaubriand, Chateau Champlain, Chateau Bonaventure); Mont Tremblant (Manoir Penatau); Garmisch Partenkirchen (Clausings Posthotel).

I've meditated about the book in Big Sur, at Ventana and at the Quail Lodge in Carmel Valley, and done so much work on my little yacht, the *Nubi II,* at the World's Fair Marina in New York and the Castaways Yacht Club, in New Rochelle, New York, and also in the marinas in Norwalk and Mystic Seaport, Connecticut; at the Shelburne Yacht Club Marina on Lake Champlain, New York; and at Norrie Yacht Basin on the Hudson, near Hyde Park.

Index

Acid/alkaline condition (pH
  factor), 13–14
Acupuncture, 120–21
Acupuncture and Your Health,
  120
Afro (natural) style, 33, 36–37,
  93
Age, hair loss and, 105, 111
Air conditioning, 24
Alberts, Howard, 43
Alexander, Dale, 122
Alexander Hair Cocktail, 122
Alexander the Great, xiv, 31
Allerest, 85
Allergic reaction, coloring and, 85
Alopecia: female androgenetic,
  112; traction, 108. *See also*
  Baldness
Amino acids, 146, 153; essential,
  146; influence on permanents,
  94; nonessential, 146
Amundsen, Roald, 138
Anagen (hair-growing stage), 104
Androgen, 111, 112, 114
Antibiotics, 110, 141
Ascorbic acid. *See under* Vitamins
Aslan, Ana, 124

Baccarat hairstyle, 49

Baden, Howard, 125
Baldness, 107–14, 115–25;
  acupuncture for, 120–21; aging
  and, 105, 111; American
  remedies, 124–25; bilobe flap,
  117–18; chemicals or drugs and,
  110; congenital, 111; hairpieces,
  119, 127–29; hair weaving, 119;
  hereditary, xv, 108, 111, 120;
  hormonal, xvi, 109, 111–12,
  113; Hungarians and, 122–23;
  infections and, 109–10; location,
  112–13; megavitamins and
  protein supplements, 121–22;
  permanent, 111–14; Rumanians
  and, 124; Russian research, 122;
  SMA profile, 113; stress and,
  110, 113; strip grafting, 118–19;
  surgical implants, 120;
  temporary, 108–10; thinning vs.,
  111; topical hormone injections,
  113–14; traction, 108;
  transplants, 115–19; traumatic,
  108–9. *See also* Fallout
Banfi, Andras ("Mr. Banfi's
  Lotion"), 122–23
Basic Four Food Plan, 132, 155
Bathing caps, 27
Beans, dried, 155, 159